Deborah

THE BIRTHING BOOK

Two Nurses Tell You How to Have an Easier Labor and Delivery

CATHERINE KEITH, R.N.
& DEBRA SPERLING, R.N.

NYT
Times
BOOKS

Published by TIMES BOOKS,
The New York Times Book Co., Inc.
130 Fifth Avenue, New York, N.Y. 10011

Published simultaneously in Canada by
Fitzhenry & Whiteside, Ltd., Toronto

Library of Congress Cataloging in Publication Data

Keith, Catherine.
The birthing book.

Includes index.
1. Childbirth. I. Sperling, Debra. II. Title.
RG525.K37 1984 618.4 83-45925
ISBN 0-8129-1112-1

Designed by Doris Borowsky

Manufactured in the United States of America

84 85 86 87 88 5 4 3 2 1

To our families, who gave us endless love and support; to our husbands, who encouraged us to pursue our dreams; and to our patients, who inspired us to write this book.

ACKNOWLEDGMENTS

We would like to take this opportunity to thank the people who assisted us on this project: thanks to Leslie Tonner, without whom this book would never have been written; to Richard Curtis, who inspired and guided the project from its inception; and to Kathleen Moloney, for her support and enthusiasm.

CONTENTS

Foreword

In this time of economic growth and stock market boom, we've become accustomed to hearing that "an educated consumer is the best customer" and "informed buyers make good buyers." So at a time of baby boom it seems appropriate to state that informed pregnant mothers make better patients.

I have seen this come true in my practice. As a New York City obstetrician, I have observed that hardly a week goes by without a patient who has just conceived (or is about to conceive!) coming into the office to interview me. The questions come fast and furious:

"Do you believe in natural childbirth?"

"Do you do episiotomies routinely?"

"Do I have to be in stirrups?"

"Does your hospital have a birthing room?"

"After delivery can I room in with the baby?"

"Do you use the fetal monitor?"

"How about I.V.'s, enemas, and shaving?"

"How many Cesarean sections do you do?"

First-time mothers-to-be have learned to ask these questions because of friends, television, or books. But even giving them the answers they want doesn't do them much good. They need to go through the nine months of pregnancy and grow with the experience, as does the baby they are carrying.

A far better concept than natural childbirth for mothers-to-be to embrace is *prepared childbirth*. Classes in prepared childbirth are given by certified childbirth educators, usually nurses or nurse midwives. They cover the physiology of pregnancy in a way that makes the pregnant couple understand the changes that are taking place throughout the pregnancy, and then they lead the couple through the various stages of childbirth. Labor is a painful experience. I know that it hurts as the uterus contracts, and I have yet to deliver a patient who has told me otherwise. And there is no question in my mind that an informed mother will have an easier time of it.

From a personal point of view, my wife and I are the proud parents of two children under two years old, and both were delivered without any anesthesia. My wife was fully prepared for the experience, fully accepting of any eventuality, and that made it easier and much more pleasant as *no self-imposed pressure* was brought to bear.

This book answers all the needs of expectant parents. It is insightful, concise, and sensitive. The authors are dedicated nurses who have shared their experience with us and have made childbirth a natural experience even when the birth process itself was not "natural." The patients who have taken their childbirth classes have been calmer, better informed, and well prepared. Most of all, they have been in greater control, so they were able to make their birth experience a joyful event.

Raymond Z. Sandler, M.D. FACOG
New York City, May 1984

THE BIRTHING BOOK

INTRODUCTION

Enlightened Childbirth: How We Can Help You

This is a good time to be having a baby. There is so much now that can be done to aid both mother and child during pregnancy and after birth. But not too many years ago the picture was quite different. Twenty or thirty years ago women vied for the honor of who was least aware during her labor and delivery. It was not uncommon to hear, "I was put to sleep, and when I woke up, they handed me my baby!" The blessing was that you did not remember a thing, and because you did not recall any pain, childbearing "didn't hurt." That was the height of modern medicine. No one worried about what effect anesthetizing the mother had on the unborn child, who absorbed much of the anesthesia as well.

Most of the recollections your mothers had of being pregnant and delivering their babies centered on their ignorance of what was happening to them. Time and again you hear, "No one ever told me what to expect. I had no idea what was coming next. They sent your father away, put me in a little room, and left. I was all alone until it was time to deliver. It seemed barbaric." Barbaric? Not at all, the ladies were told. Having babies out in the fields was barbaric.

Perhaps as a reaction to these memories, a movement toward "natural" childbirth took hold in this country in the 1960s and 1970s. Some aspects of it were the diametric opposite of those supposedly humane birthing scenes of the forties and fifties. Home births, in particular, became the modern way to do it, along with the attitude that any kind of intervention in birth was bad and made you a failure.

Now, in the 1980s, we are at a crossroads. Childbearing seems to be taking a definite turn away from the anesthetized stupor toward a more aware, informed, controlled birth. But whether this movement will take hold remains in doubt as long as there are people who espouse the view that having a baby is a feat akin to climbing Everest, one that proves one's womanliness, just as men meet challenges to test their manhood.

The book you are about to read is the product of a great deal of time and thought. The time includes our years of training in nursing school and the long days and nights spent on the labor and delivery floors. The thought involves all of the reactions and responses we have had, collectively, to the women we have seen in labor, delivering babies.

The hardest part of nursing, and of medicine in general, is seeing people suffering and feeling helpless and being unable to do anything to alleviate their pain. When we began our jobs as labor and delivery nurses, we were young (in our early twenties), enthusiastic, and energetic. We felt we could make things easier for the people we saw every day who struggled with the contractions, who were afraid of what might happen to them, and who were totally ignorant of what was going on in their bodies and of what the nurses and doctors were doing to them.

After a number of months, it became obvious that the more afraid women were, the more they suffered. The less they knew, the harder it was to bear the pain they experienced. There were some women whose experiences were far better, though. Sometimes they were students of natural childbirth teachers; other times they were women who were simply more relaxed and accepting. In their acceptance, they found a comfort the other struggling women could not discover.

It began to seem likely to us that relaxation, acceptance, and knowledge were the fundamental reasons for a woman's having a pleasant experience bearing a child. But how could we make more women better patients? How could we enable them to understand that they needed to relax and "go with the flow," comprehend their situation and accept it? There was only one answer: we had to teach. We had to tell them what we had learned as nurses in labor and delivery.

And so our classes began—four or five pregnant women accompanied by husbands and coaches, meeting over a period of six weeks, learning what they were going to face. We discussed everything from an uncomplicated vaginal birth with no anesthesia to the complications of an emergency Cesarean section. We brought in photographs, charts, and instruments. We included a hospital tour of the labor and delivery suite and maternity floor, pointing out the places they would be, showing them exactly what the nurses and doctors did. There would be no surprises for our students.

And the results? The women in our classes have had a lower percentage of births with anesthesia than the norm. And those who did have Cesarean sections, augmented labor, and epidurals did not suffer from the fairly common attacks of guilt women have because they did not go "natural." We make the women in our classes feel that their health and the health of their babies come first. We have no bias against Cesareans or anesthesia. Cesareans can save babies' lives, and anesthesia can transform an unpleasant childbirth experience into a pleasant one. We cover these subjects in depth so that no one feels she is being pushed into something she doesn't understand.

We have often been told that we should write a book, but somehow, with our jobs and classes and after-work studies toward advanced nursing degrees, we were afraid we'd never find the time. But now we have been able to translate our work into this guide to prepared childbirth, which contains material from our classes as well as other information gathered from our years of experience "on the floor."

It's all here: chapters on relaxation, breathing techniques, exercises, labor, delivery, anesthesia and analgesia, hospital procedures, problems and complications, Cesarean section, postpartum recovery, and answers to all the questions—no matter how outrageous or trivial they may seem—you might possibly ask on the subject of labor and delivery. We have discussed every subject as honestly as we can, because we believe that by knowing everything that can possibly happen to you, you will have a better labor and delivery.

This is not a book about pregnancy. We do not cover conception, diet, maternity wardrobes, morning sickness, and other topics. We do include information on doctors and midwives, doctors' visits, and exercising. But we have written what is primarily a childbirth book, told from the perspective of nurses.

What we teach and what we're writing about here is not what is generally referred to as natural childbirth. Natural childbirth has come to mean childbirth without any interference. What is being discussed is *prepared* childbirth, or what we like to call enlightened childbirth. It has less to do with *how* you have your baby and more to do with knowing everything possible that can happen to you while you are having your baby. It means acknowledging the best and the worst that could happen, what can go right and what could go wrong, and knowing that if things don't go the way you had planned (if you turn out to have an emergency Cesarean, for example), you're still as prepared as if you'd had a vaginal birth.

It means teaching your coach to help you; it means using relaxation and breathing as a form of prophylaxis. Above all, enlightened childbirth means an emphasis on the goal: labor and delivery are a small part of the role of parent. Childbirth should be an event that brings you and the baby's father closer together as a couple. And of course, the ultimate goal is a healthy mother and healthy baby.

Of course you're afraid of what will happen. People are always afraid of the unknown. It is the job of enlightened childbirth—our job—to bring you out of that dark room and into a bright place, where you can learn all about what will happen to you. It's not just being awake and aware that are important but being part of the process as well. Preparation cuts down the fear and the pain, and it will make the birth of your baby an event that will be a positive start for your new family.

We give more extensive information than most books on Cesareans, on anesthesia, and on problem labors. We put you in the delivery room, on the operating table, in the labor room, telling you exactly what the experience will be like so you know precisely what to expect. We take your husband/coach aside and give him or her tips on how to help you during your labor. And we tell you how to apply flexibility and common sense to your breathing and relaxation techniques, so that you can be the best-prepared patient possible.

CHAPTER ONE

You Have to Love It: Life on the Labor/Delivery Floor

We are often asked by the people in our classes what it's like to be a labor and delivery nurse. We glance at each other with exhaustion, for how can we explain in the little bit of time available to us what the heights of exhilaration and the depths of despair can be like all in one workday? We can speak of the long hours, the exhaustion, the mess, the unpredictability, the physical and emotional drain, which are constant, but somehow it's not enough. "You have to love it," we say. "You have to *really* love it."

Nursing in labor and delivery is a nursing of extremes. There is no constant by which you can set your body clock. It seems we're either bored to tears by a slow day or running so fast we have no time to eat, drink, or go to the bathroom. We think we've seen everything, and then something wonderful or terrible happens.

There is no "typical" day on the labor and delivery floor, but perhaps we can construct one to give you an idea of what it's like.

There are three shifts: day (from 7:00 A.M. to 3:30 P.M.), evening (3:00 P.M. to 11:30 P.M.), and night (11:15 P.M. to 7:15 A.M.). Nurses who arrive at 7:00 A.M. for the day shift receive a report from the night staff on what has occurred and who is in labor. Once the report is completed, nurses on duty are assigned to the labor rooms or birthing room. In addition to floor duties, on weekday mornings there are usually one or two elective Cesarean sections scheduled. Two nurses are assigned to assist these procedures, which begin around 8:00 A.M. One serves as a scrub nurse to assist the doctor during the surgery, and the other is a circulating nurse who takes care of the newborn baby and assists the anesthesiologist, among other functions.

There is also an average of one or two inductions taking place each day. Induced patients must have a nurse present at all times to monitor their progress.

If a nurse is not supervising an induction or assisting in the operating room, she may be with a patient in labor in her assigned room (or, on the busiest days, helping out with any and all patients on the floor). A nurse can be seeing a pregnant woman *not* in labor who has come to the hospital with a nonrelated complaint. For example, labor and delivery nurses will be sent a pregnant woman who is having an asthma attack.

There may also be a patient on the floor in premature labor. The nurse is also responsible for attending patients in the recovery room, where the women are sent after delivery. At the same time, she will have to assist the five or six pregnant women sent to the floor each day for what are known as nonstress tests.

If this doesn't sound like too much already, the nurses must also hang intravenous bottles for laboring women, administer enemas, shave patients, bring bedpans, bring food trays to women who have delivered, act as a labor coach for women whose coaches have panicked or failed to show up or left the room, and, if no nurse's aides are available, they must clean up the delivery room following a birth. There are days when things are so busy that the nurses go from one delivery to another, from one patient to another, with scarcely time to breathe. That is the time when the nurses most appreciate a couple doing well with prepared childbirth so that the presence of a nurse in constant attendance isn't necessary.

"We're psychiatrists, maids, social workers, dietitians, cleaning ladies, labor coaches, husbands, doctors. We're everything and anything," the nurses say. You can see why you have to love it.

Why would anyone choose labor and delivery nursing? The nurses agree that it's a more independent form of nursing than most other areas. We do get to make decisions. And we get to take part in one of the most exciting and meaningful experiences you could possibly have on earth. Most of the nurses have drawers full of letters, photographs, and cards sent by grateful patients. And when someone who has taken childbirth preparation in our own class delivers, it is even more exciting. Labor and delivery is known as the happiest area of nursing, for it's the one with the nicest outcome. The nurses admit that they can get so involved in someone's labor that they will voluntarily stay after hours just to be present at the delivery. "You want to see someone through," they say. "You've struggled with the patient for six hours, you've even gotten up on the bed with her to help her out, she's finally fully dilated—and it's time to go home. So you stick around just a bit more." A bit more sometimes means an additional two, three, or four hours of work. But the nurses agree that it's worth it.

You need many attributes to be a labor and delivery nurse, not just an endless supply of adrenaline. You also require the following: years of experience, patience, a strong bladder, support stockings, kindness, a gentle touch, and a calm, reassuring manner. Because we are unfamiliar with the patients who come in during their labors, we have to establish a relationship with them very quickly. And for this, you need to be open, direct, and "up front."

But what about the bad times? "Sometimes it's very sad. The things that happen seem to be the saddest things that ever happened," one nurse said. It is extremely difficult to watch new mothers cry when something goes wrong. The nurses say you have to learn not to cry along with them.

Life on the labor and delivery floor can be very emotional, with feelings running close to the surface at all times. It abounds with contradictions—happiness one moment, sadness the next. The contrasts are sometimes shocking. In one room, a drug addict with needle marks in her arm can be giving birth to a screaming baby, while down the hall a woman who has had half a dozen miscarriages is having another in spite of all our efforts to save the fetus. That's the contradiction of our job, and of our day-to-day lives.

CHAPTER TWO

Yes, It Hurts: Coping With the Pain

You'll discover that being pregnant makes you fair game for the rest of the world's mothers, who are only too eager and happy to tell you what happened to them when they had their babies. You'll hear stories told in excruciating detail of how labor and delivery went. Often the sources of the worst of these tales will be your own mothers and mothers-in-law, who had their babies twenty or thirty years ago and don't realize that things are different today.

Then there are the childbirth sequences in movies and television shows, which seem to specialize in scenes of agony that last endless hours. Misinformation flies fast and furious. You hear about twilight sleep, dry births, high forceps, umbilical cords twisted around babies' necks, and women sewn up too tightly. It's enough to make you think you'll never survive. But you *will* survive. And not only will you survive, you'll be as prepared and informed as possible so that you will never have to say that you did not know what was happening to you.

Of course it hurts to have a baby. But there is plenty that you and your husband or coach can do to make childbirth a positive, enriching experience.

By now you may be wondering about what all these people—doctors, nurses, childbirth instructors, *we*—are telling you. Some of the women who will be helping you have never had children themselves; none of the men, obviously, has ever been in labor. How do they know what it's like? How can they tell you what to expect? How many times have we women been examined by a male doctor and told, "This won't hurt," only to hit the ceiling a few seconds later? Is it the same with having babies? Are veterans the only fair judges?

In many ways, women who have borne children are at a certain disadvantage as far as teaching and explaining about labor. Their own experiences have colored their viewpoints. If their labor was especially easy, they'll probably tone down their warnings about pain. If it was the worst, they may exaggerate their picture of labor in general. The best judges may well be those people who haven't had children. From their own experience, nurses and doctors, who have seen thousands of babies being delivered, can extract what is probably the median or moderate view of what is going on and present it in a way that will prepare you for both the best and the worst.

What all this means is that you must not discount the testimony of the professionals, even though they may be lacking the primary experience. They know a great deal about what's going to happen to you.

Which brings us to the subject of pain. Pain is the great barrier, that seemingly insurmountable wall you imagine you must scale before someone places a baby in your arms. It's the no-man's-land everyone fears, because it is regarded as a kind of ultimate test. It is also one of the hardest things to measure, because so much about pain is subjective, dependent on your cultural conditioning, your past experiences, and your particular threshold. For instance, a woman who has never experienced a severe menstrual pain in her life may find the onset of labor more painful than her friend who has had to cope with terrible menstrual cramps. A long, drawn-out labor might be less painful than a short, intense one with harder contractions.

One thing is important to remember: after childbirth, few women can recollect the pain exactly. Even monitoring the contractions, which gives evidence of duration and frequency, does not accurately reflect how much it hurts. With all these subjective aspects to keep in mind, it must seem impossible to determine how much childbirth actually hurts.

That is why many prepared childbirth classes don't discuss pain. The instructors speak of "waves" sweeping over your body; the books talk about "flowing" with the contractions and about experiencing some "discomfort"; but pain is a four-letter word that is rarely mentioned.

This is where some frankness and honesty ought to come in. It *does* hurt to have a baby. How much it hurts varies from woman to woman, but the woman who has not been told to expect pain may be hard pressed to describe her contractions as "waves" when the going gets rough. You may be one of the lucky ones, with a quick, briefly intense labor that's over in a matter of hours, but if you're not, you'll feel even worse if you're not ready for pain.

You have to talk about the pain: talk to your doctor, to your midwife, to your childbirth instructor, to the other couples in your childbirth classes. By facing the fact that labor will be painful, you will then come to understand that you can do something about it. By learning how to relax, how to breathe properly, and how to respond to coaching, you can diminish the effect of the pain.

Remember that when your labor begins, you will most likely be at home. You won't be going to the hospital until your labor is well under way, if everything is going normally. And when you get to the hospital, it's likely too that you will not receive any anesthesia immediately. Preparing properly for childbirth will aid you each step of the way, so that at all times, you, not the pain, are in control.

But how, you ask, can you be in control in the atmosphere of a hospital labor and delivery suite? Everyone knows how rigid most hospitals are about rules and regulations, how unyielding and inflexible many doctors and nurses can seem in stressful situations. How can it be different during childbirth?

The answer is that your *attitude* can make it work. There are six basic things we'd like you to learn right away and remember.

1. Times have changed. Many of the old negative attitudes toward intervention, especially toward Cesarean section and anesthesia, were based on procedures that are now out of date. Women's fears were grounded in the very real facts that a Cesarean was major abdominal surgery, that you were put to sleep during one, that even husbands trained in natural childbirth techniques were barred from delivery rooms, and that the anesthesia used had a less than benign effect on the newborn baby.

Today, Cesarean mothers are awake during their surgery; they are given, for the most part, regional anesthesia; the surgery is far simpler; and, in many hospitals, if application is made in advance, fathers are permitted in the operating room. Anesthesia given today is no longer the strong sleeping drug administered years ago but more likely the simpler epidural, which is given gradually until a localized numbing takes effect below the waist.

2. Fear makes pain worse. Women who don't know what's going to happen to them will have a much harder time controlling the pain, because their fear will make that pain much worse. Knowing what to expect—even if you have to face an emergency—can make a big difference. And learning to relax can enable you to tolerate the pain more effectively and handle it well. That is far better than freezing with fear, tensing up, thrashing around, and losing control.

3. It helps to be prepared. Your doctor or midwife will be happy to discuss all of your choices with you ahead of time. Since you have appointments on a regular basis, it is possible to set aside a bit of time each month to raise some of the questions about your birthing experience then. Be conscientious about asking these questions. Keep a pad and pencil on your bedside table and in your purse. Write down *anything* you want to know about, no matter how trivial. If it makes a difference to you that you may be allowed to keep your wedding ring on during delivery, then by all means ask your doctor if that is okay. (It is.) You'd be surprised what many expectant mothers want to know, from questions about wearing makeup ("Can I leave my nail polish on?") to queries about enemas, stitches, shaving, and other hospital procedures.

Doctors and hospitals have become far more flexible over the last half-dozen years, and if you ask, you may discover that your doctor won't insist on doing something you might find uncomfortable *if* your labor is proceeding without problems. Or your doctor may give such a good explanation for some things that bother you that you may accept them more willingly. You'll never know, however, unless you ask.

4. You are not alone. Childbirth is no longer a case of that poor woman shut inside a room by herself, struggling with things she doesn't understand. Birth is a joint effort, a joint pulling together of mother, father or coach, labor nurse, and doctor or midwife. And this is a good time to point out that you may choose anyone to be your coach; it doesn't always have to be the husband and father. Your coach can be your boyfriend, your best girl friend, your sister, your aunt, your mother, your childbirth teacher, or, simply, your labor nurse. Labor nurses who are prepared childbirth instructors have seen more women than they can count through their labors and deliveries, even at times giving unprepared women quick bedside courses in how to relax and breathe properly during contractions.

5. You can always ask for anesthesia. Learning about prepared childbirth, learning the exercises and the breathing, attending classes and participating fully in the program, does *not* mean that you are committed to having your baby without anesthesia. On the contrary, anesthesia and pain-reducing drugs are fine and can be used; it's just helpful to remember that they will not be used at the pain of the first contraction. It will always help to know what is going to happen regardless of which path you choose.

6. The doctor makes a difference. Make sure your doctor suits your needs. Discuss everything ahead of time and make certain that he will not push you toward using anesthesia if you don't want to, or try to influence you to reject any interference. If you disagree strongly and you feel there is no compromise, try to find someone more compatible. Pregnancy makes all women a great deal more sensitive than they are normally, and it is especially important that you feel reassured by your physician. Don't allow any of your fears or questions to be dismissed. Physicians and midwives are customarily very obliging about discussing any procedures with you as far in advance as you like. So don't be afraid to speak up at your first or second appointment and find out how he feels about childbirth with or without interference. Your feeling of confidence in your doctor will assist you greatly during labor and delivery, adding to that important sense of being in control.

CHAPTER THREE

Your Best Friend: All About Coaches

One of the most widely recognized aspects of prepared childbirth is the presence of the coach, usually the husband, during labor and delivery. But this image isn't always a positive one. In fact, one of the stumbling blocks to getting couples into childbirth education classes is the reluctance of the husband to *be* the coach.

"I'll throw up," they tell us. "I can't stand the sight of blood." Or, "I don't want to see my wife in pain." Or, "What do I do if she screams?"

Many pregnant women call us up before their classes are scheduled to start to ask what we can do about the reluctance of their husbands to participate. Just get them to the first class, we urge them. Then we'll take over.

And what is it that makes the difference between someone who turns green at the mention of contractions, placenta, episiotomy, and someone who cannot stop talking about how *he* was there and the doctor let *him* cut the cord?

The difference is knowing he's needed.

And what we tell the coaches is that they are truly necessary and as important a part in this entire process as the woman having her baby. In fact, she couldn't do it without *him*. Coaches are indispensable, the most important key to the success of prepared childbirth.

The coach is, after the pregnant woman, the most important person in the labor room. He's the co-captain of your team, the one person who can speak for you if you cannot make it clear what you want. You've learned everything together; you've discussed everything with your coach ahead of time; and all decisions during labor and delivery should be cleared with *both* of you. For the coach prepares as you prepare; coaches know as much as the woman in labor. In fact, they sometimes know more, for many a laboring woman loses her cool and concentration and forgets what she has learned; the coach is there to get her back on the track. And a coach is the single most important source of support in this endeavor. A coach is not there simply to watch; he is there to participate.

Before we discuss more about what coaches do, perhaps we should say a word about who coaches are. In most instances, the coach is the woman's husband. If the couple isn't married, the baby's father is an appropriate coach if he is interested and involved in the pregnancy.

But the role is not limited to men. Your mother, sister, aunt, mother-in-law, or best friend can all be candidates for the job. Several women have turned up at the hospital with their own fathers as coaches, though Dad chose to wait outside the delivery room for the baby's birth. If all the people you ask cannot attend the childbirth classes or read this book, or if you've just moved to a new town and know no one, you should understand that you can study and use prepared childbirth techniques alone; it's just harder that way than with a coach. But in most hospitals, once you're in labor, there will be labor nurses to cheer you on and assist you and serve as stand-ins for the coach.

The coach learns along with the pregnant woman, attending childbirth classes, visiting the hospital, studying the same written materials. Persuade your coach to read this book with you if you can; if nothing else, get him to read this chapter and the various "memos to the coach" that are included in the body of most chapters. These summarize the most important points of coaching and provide a list of tips on how to do the job well.

In addition to observing and studying, the coach also learns *how* to do everything as well. He practices relaxation techniques, switching places with his partner so as to learn how to recognize tension and how a relaxed muscle feels. He learns the breathing exercises and again participates in practicing the techniques. In fact, in our classes we also suggest that the coach get down on the floor and practice the pushing exercises, even though he lacks the same set of muscles with which to push. By experiencing the physical methods together, the couple learns to work interchangeably. It helps him to understand what *she* is going through; and it helps her to understand *his* role. During childbirth, this can lead to a better bond between the pair. There is more trust and there is more openness. You have to be willing to criticize each other and to stop the other person if something is being done wrong. You have to know how hard to press on someone's back should most of the labor take place there, or how gently to stroke a neck and shoulders in order to help relieve the tension.

Practicing together strengthens the bond between the pregnant woman and her coach. It may be easy to say, "We're both really tired tonight, so let's skip the practicing just this once and go to sleep early," but you aren't doing anyone a favor by skipping a practice session. Practicing is the most important thing you'll be doing during the last weeks of the pregnancy. It must be emphasized that by shirking practice, you are undermining the entire program and cannot expect it to provide you with enough help when you need it. Only through practice will you gain the confidence that will make your childbirth experience a better one for all concerned—you, the coach, and the baby.

But it's not only homework, this required practice of relaxation, exercise, and breathing. You are also getting used to working with the one person who can give you the words of encouragement and the help that will be so crucial during labor. If a woman does not remember what she is supposed to do, if she does the breathing wrong, if she tenses when she should be relaxing, if she forgets to use a focal point or to take a cleansing breath or to switch to a more comfortable position, then everything she has learned isn't going to help. And if she does it right, the coach will know how important his presence can be. Do the exercises, learn everything together so you can be truly together—in control, a team—when the time comes.

Of course, almost everyone awaiting a baby is nervous, and the coach's nervousness is compounded by his fear that he will make a complete fool of himself. Expectant fathers are known to be jittery; the added responsibilities of coaching may seem overwhelming. But perhaps we can add a few things here that might make the prospect seem less threatening.

First of all, there are some hospitals that require fathers and coaches to show a certificate proving they have completed a prepared childbirth course in order to be admitted into the delivery room. Find out ahead of time if your hospital has this requirement. If so, enroll in the classes, get the necessary certificate, and pack it with your hospital things. This will alleviate one of the most upsetting fears for all concerned—the fear that you will be separated from your husband and his fear that he will be shut away from you—when you are in pain and need him.

If you know in advance you are having a Cesarean section, your hospital may allow your coach into the delivery room. This possibility must be checked in advance. But remember that it applies for the most part to those Cesareans that are scheduled, not emergency surgery. It should also be mentioned that if a coach shows signs of squeamishness ahead of time—if he gags and starts to retch when your water is broken, or if he is sweaty and shaking—he may be denied admittance to the delivery room. If, in some cases, there are potential problems with the delivery, he may not be allowed in either. This is just to give you a few guidelines on what to expect in terms of being in the delivery room. Once you are there, however, you're on your own!

The behavior of fathers in the delivery room also covers a wide range of types. Often we'll know ahead of time just how a father will react. Some men turn pale during their wives' epidurals, when a small needle is administered to a spot on the back. It hardly hurts her at all, but watch his face! Others begin shaking or vomiting on the way to the delivery room. There are instances when the reaction can't be predicted: fathers faint in the delivery room not from the sight of blood but because the anticipated baby turned out to be twins. And there was a case of one stubborn father who stood between his wife's legs as she lay on the delivery table and refused to step aside for the doctor.

Here's a guide to recognizable types of fathers/coaches that covers just about the entire panorama of strange delivery-room behavior:

1. The Directors. Some fathers bring several cameras into the delivery room, leave their empty film boxes on the delivery table, set their flashes wrong, use the wrong lens, mess up all their shots, and generally miss the entire birth.

2. The Would-be Doctors. They have obviously studied up. "Will you be doing a medialateral incision?" they ask professionally. "Ah, now I see the caput crowning," they observe. Very medical comments issue forth throughout the entire birth.

3. The Zombies. They forget their role, forget where they are, forget what is going on, and simply stand there, in shock, and stare.

4. The Inquiring Reporters. They ask questions. "Why are you doing this?" "Why do you hold her leg up that way?" "Why does the baby look so wet?" "Why does my wife seem uncomfortable?" "How long will this take?" "How soon will it all be over?" "Is what you're doing really necessary?"

5. The Quick-change Artists. There are fathers who wait until the last second to change into their scrub suits and then hurry so they won't miss anything in the delivery room—with surprising results. Some come running out half-naked, without their pants. Some pull the scrub suits on over their shirts and pants, leaving their long sleeves hanging out. Some forget to keep their shoes and socks on, as instructed, and run out in bare feet. Most wear their masks wrong, inside out or upside down, or wear the mask below their noses instead of over them. But all the fathers are proud to have been in the delivery room, and some wear their masks for hours afterward, a symbol of what *they've* been through.

CHAPTER FOUR

The Maternity Establishment: Health-Care Professionals

Now that you have a coach and understand how he'll help you, it would be a good idea to discuss some of the other people who'll be instrumental in the birth of your child, and to talk about some of the things you'll be doing in connection with your pregnancy.

By the time you have bought this book, you should have a doctor selected to deliver your baby, or you may have chosen a midwife practicing at a local hospital. In either case, you'll be paying this professional monthly visits, and at the end of your pregnancy, weekly ones, so you'll get to know your doctor or midwife quite well. If you have a strong difference of opinion with this professional on how your pregnancy is going to be managed or any serious problem of communication, you can switch to someone else. Remember that you are the most important person to be considered and that it's crucial for you to be secure in your choice of doctor. Many patients are concerned with hurting the doctor's feelings, but this should not stand in your way if there is a serious reason to change physicians (not just that you don't like the color of his socks, for example).

Plan what you'll ask during a doctor's visit. As we have mentioned, you should be writing down any questions you have about your pregnancy. Take them with you to your office visits. You'd be amazed at how many women become completely tongue-tied or forgetful in the presence of their doctor. It's a frequent complaint; "I forgot to ask the doctor something," they explain when they call back an hour later. And of course, the answer they get on the phone is never as satisfactory as it would have been in person, in the physician's reassuring presence.

No question is too trivial. You are the keeper of your body; you know it better than anyone. Odd feelings or aches and pains, however small, should be mentioned. Any fears or fantasies that trouble you should be raised. The nice thing about obstetricians is that they genuinely care about pregnant women and have a very broad-minded approach to their treatment. You aren't being indulged as a foolish person when you bring up what's bothering you; you'll be listened to as someone important. Pregnancies are their business.

If you've been to your doctor already, then you have some idea what office visits are like. For those who haven't been yet, the routine is pretty much the same from doctor to doctor. First of all, if you're seeing someone with his own practice, then each time you visit, that doctor will be there. If he goes on vacation, he will get someone to cover for him, but generally, you'll be with one person from start to finish.

Should your doctor be in partnership with another physician, you'll alternate visits from one to the other in some cases. The doctor on call will be the one who delivers your baby. This is a very nice situation, as you'll come to know both doctors well and won't feel uncomfortable if one or the other is on when you go into labor. Some partnerships, however, work like single practices in that you see only one doctor throughout your pregnancy, with the other serving as backup in case your physician isn't available. In group practices the same conditions apply. Either you switch around and see whichever doctor is in the office that day, or you stick with one and may get another when your time to deliver comes. You should decide ahead of time which situation will be most comfortable for you. Some women prefer only one doctor; others like the security of feeling there's a team working for them.

During a typical office visit, your doctor's nurse or assistant will ask you to leave a urine sample, which is tested for excess sugar or protein. Excess sugar might indicate that the woman is developing what is known as gestational diabetes, a form of diabetes that can occur during pregnancy and disappears once the baby is delivered. Excess protein might mean the patient is developing toxemia, another disease of pregnancy, which is treated by bed rest and closer medical supervision. Toxemia—or preeclampsia, as it is sometimes called—is a condition in which the woman retains a great deal of water (edema). This is signaled by a sudden weight gain and marked swelling and is accompanied by high blood pressure. Neither of these problems is life-threatening for you or the baby if you have good medical care. And with the monthly urine test, you are being constantly supervised.

The doctor will then see you and each month will perform the same ritual. You'll be weighed in; your blood pressure will be checked; and you will be examined (most often externally). Around the twelfth to the sixteenth week of your pregnancy, the doctor will try to listen to the beating of the fetal heart. He has a special stethoscope for that purpose, with a metal piece that fits over his head; it can pick up sounds a regular stethoscope cannot. You may be permitted to listen to the heartbeat as well, and if you'd like, you can bring in your husband, your mother, or anyone else you'd like to hear the sound of the unborn baby.

Customarily, the doctor will ask you back into his office from the examining room in order to have a short consultation. Here he will give you any instructions necessary for the next month of your pregnancy, he'll answer your questions, he'll discuss what you may expect in the next few months. This is the time to pull out that pad with the questions written down on it.

There is something you ought to be aware of in connection with visits to doctors or midwives, and that is that the monthly visits are extremely short. Sometimes they only last about five minutes. You may feel, Hey, I'm paying all this money and that's all the time I get? Or, How can the doctor possibly know what's going on, or spot what's going wrong in so short a time? The answer is first of all that pregnant women are, for the most part, *well* women. You're not sick if you're pregnant. For many women, it's the healthiest time of their lives. They're eating well, getting a lot of sleep, doing some exercise, taking good care of themselves. Second, the doctor is so familiar with the norms that there really doesn't have to be a lot of time expended in the examination; he can spot a problem at once. If you've chosen your doctor with care and if you are satisfied with his reputation, you can be assured that you and your baby are in good hands.

Visits to a midwife are just the same, with the exception of a few visits paid during your pregnancy to a doctor who works with the midwife. This is to make certain that there are no conditions that might require delivery by the doctor, such as those that result in Cesarean section, which will be discussed in a later chapter. The doctor just wants to make certain that everything is going well. These checkups are in addition to the care you'll be receiving directly from the midwife herself.

Many patients choose the nurse-midwife to find a birth experience they feel will meet their needs. The trend for labor and delivery nurses to become midwives is a logical extension of the more involved role of labor nurse. But instead of stepping away as the patient is ready to deliver to assist the doctor, the midwife delivers the baby. The midwife can make all decisions on her own, and except for such procedures as a forceps delivery or a Cesarean section, she can see the patient through a complete labor and delivery. Most midwives are required to have some experience as labor and delivery nurses. Patients who want to have their babies delivered by midwives in a nurse-midwife program generally have to be those women who are not expected to have a problem pregnancy. Anything not part of the normal antepartum, labor, or delivery becomes the province of the obstetrician.

Many hospitals are now participating in the midwifery program or contemplating such participation, because it removes a great burden from the physician to have normal pregnancies taken care of by the midwife. It is also far less expensive to be in a program with midwives, and, for the woman interested in prepared childbirth, it can be a pleasant and safe alternative. For the nurses who become deeply involved in teaching childbirth classes and who feel that prepared patients can have easier labors and deliveries, becoming a midwife is indeed the next natural step. It can prove to be the most satisfying outlet for an involved, committed labor nurse.

Along with this new relationship between nurse-midwives and patients, there is also a different relationship taking place between patients and doctors. Prepared childbirth has not only helped to create a demand for more nurse-midwives, it has also helped to create doctors' patients who are more educated, who demand more information, and who want to know more about all the options available. They are searching for doctors who meet their needs. In response to this, doctors have had to become more responsive to their patients. In fact, many refer to patients as clients and treat them with more of a businesslike manner than the old "father/obstetrician–daughter/pregnant woman" relationship dictated. Patients are now picking and choosing among the doctors; they want—indeed they require—a doctor who understands all aspects of prepared childbirth.

The next health-care professionals you may meet are the prepared childbirth educators. And please, don't shy away from prepared childbirth classes. No one will force you to have your baby without anesthesia, or to do something you don't want to do. Take an opportunity to learn everything you need to have a better labor and delivery; use what you learn in this book, and then apply it to the lessons in your prepared childbirth classes. For your coach, who may already be balking at reading any books, childbirth classes are invaluable for learning to recognize what is going on and coming to understand what's happening in each stage of labor. Don't rely on simply reading what to do; your book learning should be supplemented by at least one or two and if possible five or six classes to cover all the basics. At minimum, you should be taught to breathe correctly under the supervision of a proper teacher. Practice in front of the experts before you make your debut. Then, in the privacy of your home, when the moment arrives, you and your coach won't panic about what to do. It will be second nature by then.

Ask your doctor or midwife where you can take your classes. They are customarily given for women in their sixth or seventh month of pregnancy. You can also contact the hospital at which you will be giving birth for information on childbirth classes in your area. Or there may be a childbirth preparation center advertising in the Yellow Pages. Most classes aren't very expensive and require just a few hours of your time over a period of several weeks. They will make a great deal of difference in your confidence level, and in labor, confidence counts.

What are childbirth classes like? We can tell you about our own.

Everyone who comes to the classes is nervous, so we generally open with a round-robin discussion in which we ask the couples who come why they decided to take classes. Here are some of the answers we've been given:

"My wife made me come."

"I [the husband] want to be in the delivery room."

"I [the wife] want to be more informed; I want to know what's going on."

"My doctor said I should."

"It seemed like something I could do to help myself in my pregnancy."

"Everyone else is doing it."

"I don't know why I'm here."

"I'm afraid [of labor, of delivery, of pain, of Cesarean sections, of anesthesia, of doctors, of hospitals, of babies, of enemas, of prepping, etc.]."

Some of the reasons for coming don't seem very satisfactory at all, but the important thing is that couples do come. Once they're in that room, we can begin to show them why it's a good thing that they did decide to come, for whatever reason they had.

Another good reason to come to class, although it is one nobody realizes until after the classes are over, is that the class becomes a place where women whose babies are due in the same time frame can share their aches and pains and problems and fears with other women in exactly the same position. As one mother-to-be said to us, "I can't talk to my friends who aren't pregnant. They don't want to hear about my chafing thighs and my heartburn. Here I find out that someone else has lower back trouble or varicose veins, and somehow my problems aren't all that bad anymore." A natural spin-off of childbirth classes is that friendships have begun among the couples that last a long time after the babies are born. You naturally need the company of other pregnant women; don't feel shy about it. It's true that sometimes they are the only ones who'll understand.

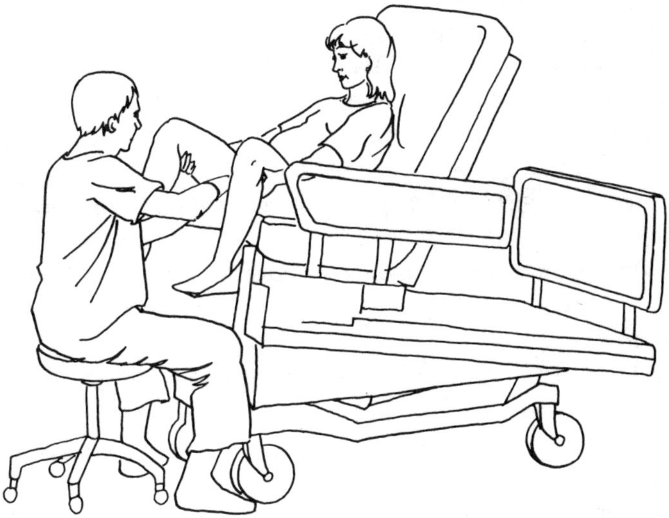

Figure 1: The birthing bed, delivery position

Childbirth classes customarily begin when the pregnant woman is at or close to the thirtieth week of her pregnancy. Many sessions meet five or six times, with each class covering a specific topic. Some childbirth instructors also include a hospital tour as the final meeting. The couples are shown the labor and delivery rooms; monitors and other instruments are pointed out to them; birthing rooms, if present at their hospital, are visited; and finally, the group makes a trip to the postpartum floor for a glance at the babies in the nursery. For women entering their final weeks of pregnancy, the visit can be inspirational. It also prevents that last-minute "I don't know what's going to happen to me" feeling by preparing the woman for what to expect in terms of a physical setup. Women in labor feel far better knowing just what's in store, rather than having any surprises sprung on them at the last moment.

There is a decision about your hospital care that you may be asked to make in advance, and that is whether you want to deliver in a birthing room (if your hospital has one). In the birthing room, you labor and deliver in the same bed. There are special birthing beds or chairs in which the bottom will drop away and leave your perineum right on the edge of the bed. Birthing beds (*Figure 1*) are designed for comfort in many positions during labor, including sitting up, sitting with the back elevated at an angle, lying down with the bottom under the buttocks raised, or lying with the legs elevated. Birthing rooms are reserved for complication- and anesthesia-free labors within the hospital setting. They are usually the rooms with the homiest atmosphere: prints on the wall, an easy chair for the coach, sometimes a television or telephone. You can find out all about the birthing room if your hospital has one, so you'll know just what to expect there. One laboring woman at our hospital stopped in her tracks at the door of our birthing room and refused to go any farther. "Where," she demanded, "is the wall-to-wall carpeting? My doctor promised me there was going to be a wall-to-wall carpet!"

In a labor room, you may share space with another woman in labor, though women are not doubled up unless it's absolutely necessary because of space. When the baby's birth is imminent, you'll be taken to the delivery room for the birth.

In order to compare birthing rooms with labor and delivery rooms, the hospital tour can be particularly useful. If your childbirth classes do not include such a tour, contact the hospital where you are going to give birth. Many hospitals now offer the mothers-to-be a look inside the birthing facilities, and it will certainly help you make a choice to have the setting shown to you ahead of time. Also, there will be fewer hospital fears along with all the other tensions you can experience at the onset of labor. Many women in labor are well and for the most part young, and most have never been inside a hospital in their lives. The delivery room, with its surgical equipment neatly laid out and its huge overhead arc lights, can seem less threatening if you see it when you're standing up.

You will not find any information here on home births, since we don't recommend them; we feel that a hospital is the best setting for childbirth. We have seen what can go wrong and feel that the best choice is still the place that offers the latest in medical and surgical care.

And finally, there is one thing you ought to know

about most health-care professionals. They've seen just about everything and anything, and most have remarkably good senses of humor. You would, too, if you'd witnessed some of the things we've seen. As an example, take this little family scene that took place very early one morning in the birthing room.

Nurses passing the birthing room were astonished to hear strange sounds issuing from behind the door. A woman moaned, then said, "Ahhhh, ohhhh, yes, I feel it, yes." The nurses thought the couple was having sex. Anxious to advise them not to during labor, one of the nurses entered the room and found the husband standing between his wife's spreadeagled legs, moving his hands in a hocus-pocus, magicianlike, coaxing gesture toward her vagina, then away from her vagina, saying, "Come out, Derek. Open up like a flower and pass through. You can do it! We all have faith in you. Don't be afraid."

The nurse, feeling like a character from the movie *Hospital*, tiptoed quietly out of the room.

CHAPTER FIVE

The Four Commandments: The Fundamentals of Technique

There are four basic principles to remember when you learn your relaxation, your exercises, and your breathing. We call them the *fundamentals of technique*. They must be applied to every simulated contraction, to every practice session, and eventually to each real contraction in labor. They must be absorbed and remembered so that they become second nature to you. When labor begins, you won't have to think about them; they'll simply be there.

1. Choose a Comfortable Position.

Whenever you practice, no matter what it is you're doing—relaxation, breathing, exercising—find a comfortable position. If you are uncomfortable, everything is going to hurt more. Being comfortable decreases stress, distraction, and muscle tension. Never lie flat on your back (except in the one or two exercises calling for this position). In labor, the weight of the baby pressing on your major blood vessels will constrict the flow of blood to your heart. The baby also presses on your lower back, which is extremely uncomfortable. If you wish to lie down on your back, prop yourself up at a 45 degree angle with some pillows. A preferred position is to lie on your side; many women are very comfortable in labor that way. You may also sit straight up, Indian style, with your legs crossed in what is called the tailor sit. Experiment with various positions so that if you are uncomfortable when your contractions start, you'll automatically know which position you should get into to be most comfortable.

2. Find a Focal Point.

Select one unmoving object at eye level or below on which you will concentrate so as to divert your attention from the contraction. Your brain, on receiving this strong stimulus, will be less receptive to the pain. The object should be at eye level or below so that you won't have to strain your head and neck to see it and thus add to your body's tension. You do not have to have the same focal point all the time, but you must never change focal points during a contraction. Choose one thing and stick to it, at least for the length of one pain. It can be anything—a doorknob, a vase, a potted plant, a piece of furniture, a picture, or a stuffed animal.

Most women find that simpler objects are easier to concentrate on; you probably should not choose a reproduction of a Jackson Pollock painting, for instance. It's too busy. Also, something with some emotional value is good, such as a snapshot of yourself and your husband. You should not get too accustomed to one focal point, however, because during labor you will have to change positions, and you may not be able to keep one object in view the entire time. Laboring women have turned up at the hospital with all sorts of things. One woman brought in an infant's christening dress, all elaborate lace and ruffles, but there was no place to put it. An ingenious nurse finally hung it from an I.V. pole. Another woman came puffing and panting in the door. Following her was her husband, who was dragging a huge, nearly life-sized stuffed bear named Seymour. "We're in labor," the husband announced as he propped the bear up so that his wife could focus on it.

Focal points (of any kind) serve to increase your concentration and lower your distraction, and you will find them invaluable aids to your breathing and relaxation. They will be discussed further in Chapter 8, which deals with breathing.

3. Take Deep, Cleansing Breaths.

A deep breath—inhalation and exhalation—should be taken at the beginning and the end of each and every contraction. They should be practiced religiously so they become automatic, during exercise and relaxation as well. The deep breath should be taken in through the nose and let out through the mouth. The breath should be slow, very concentrated and exaggerated, about twice as slow as a normal breath. As you inhale a long, prolonged breath, you will be signaling yourself to begin your concentration. As you exhale slowly and deeply, you should allow your whole body to go limp, to "flow out" along with the breath. This will be your signal to relax.

Deep breaths serve several functions, all of them important either physically or psychologically. First, by breathing deeply, you are oxygenating yourself and your baby at a critical moment when, during a contraction, you are both being deprived of extra oxygen. Second, in using the proper breathing techniques you may find yourself a bit short of breath by the end of a contraction, and the deep breath will help you regain your equilibrium. Third, the deep breaths are an important part of your psychological conditioning, because the inhaling and exhaling signal the beginning and the end of a contraction. This enables you to treat each contraction as a separate entity, one at a time. And finally, the deep breaths serve as signals to your coach that the contraction has begun and has ended. As the coach's role is discussed later on, you will see how important these signals are.

4. Practice Both Verbal and Nonverbal Cues.

These refer to the words, signals, or touches used to elicit a particular response. They will help the woman in labor by reminding her of specific responses she has learned, and they are an invaluable part of the coaching process. One important verbal cue is the phrase *contraction begins*. When you are practicing with simulated contractions, this phrase becomes the signal to start concentrating on the focal point, relaxing the muscles of your body, and begin your breathing. Without the stimulus of the actual pain of the contraction, the words serve as the signal to produce the conditioned response. After practice, the responses to this cue should be automatic.

The same is true of the words *contraction ends*. This cue signals the period of time during which you should relax between contractions. In its way, this is as important as the proper response during the contraction, for it enables you to take a break from the work that actual labor is.

Memo to the Coach

Remember that cues to relax should be delivered in a gentle, encouraging voice, in spite of the fact that the person you're telling to relax may be flailing around. And speaking of encouragement, any kind of positive verbal reinforcement is good, as long as the woman in labor can stand listening to it. "You're doing well" or "That was terrific" are fine, unless such chatter decreases her concentration. (Labor requires so much concentration that some women reach a point where they cannot bear being spoken to, and they'll let you know. One husband, trying to be helpful, was a paragon of verbal encouragement. "Oh my little sweetie, you're so wonderful, so marvelous, you're doing so fabulously, is there anything I can do for you? Just let me know, just tell me whatever you want—" and with that, his wife looked up and said, "Will you just shut up?")

During the simulated contraction, you will also be hearing the words *contraction peaking*, approximately halfway through the exercise. During hard, active labor, these words will be spoken by the coach, as he will be able to see the peak on the monitor. When you hear him say this, you'll know that the strongest part is over and it's only going to get better. Another cue, which is obvious, is the word *relax*.

Sometimes nonverbal cues should be substituted for the verbal ones. There is stroking, used to help with relaxation, which is covered in the next chapter. There are signals that can take the place of words—holding up one, two, or three fingers to show which breathing technique to use, for instance. Or sometimes the best cues are just simple nods and smiles of encouragement.

CHAPTER SIX

"Relax, Dammit!": The Principles of Relaxation

It is not difficult to tell if a patient is having a hard time relaxing during her labor contractions. You come into the labor room and there she is, experiencing a contraction, her eyes squeezed shut, her face contorted into a grimace, her hands squeezing the rails of the bed or her husband's hands. "Ow," he yells, as she digs her nails in. Her response is to squeeze harder. The nurse approaches, and as the next contraction begins, she reaches down to try to show the patient how to assume a more relaxed position. As the nurse touches the patient, the woman grabs the nurse around her neck. The husband, now freed from the death grip, shouts, "Relax, dammit!"

Not relaxing is more than merely uncomfortable for

the people present in the labor room. It makes labor far more difficult for the woman. Tensing your body in anticipation of pain not only creates a psychological barrier to being helped; it also adds to your discomfort in a simple physical way. The uterus is a muscle, and during a contraction, much of the pain is caused by oxygen deprivation. This is similar to the effect of oxygen deprivation on the heart muscle during a heart attack. By tensing other muscles in your body, you deprive your body of oxygen and, consequently, you increase the pain.

Think of your conditioned response when you go to the dentist. You've got a big hole in your left lower molar. You're in a lot of pain, but you know that once the dentist touches you, you'll be in agony. You sit down in the chair and stare at the drill. The dentist smiles, picks up the drill, and moves it toward your mouth. What's your response? You squeeze the arms of the chair, pushing down, contracting your muscles. You are doing what you have done ever since you were a child: preparing your body for pain. This is a conditioned reflex that must be overcome; and you are about to be reconditioned.

In prepared, structured childbirth education, there is physical as well as psychological preparation. Physically, you can exercise to improve your muscle tone and to allow your body to perform at its maximum ability. Psychologically, you can undergo conditioning and learn a new form of discipline and concentration, perhaps unlike any you've ever experienced before. You will learn to alter your behavior, to change your response to discomfort and pain. You will learn to perform certain physical activities and to concentrate on other stimuli to replace the input of pain. And through practice and with motivation, this reconditioning can be accomplished in a matter of weeks.

By not relaxing during a contraction, you are forgetting that in a matter of seconds (60, on the average), the contraction increases, levels off, decreases, then goes away entirely. Dealing with the pain in 60-second intervals would make it much easier to get through, whereas fighting it can make it seem much longer.

Try this simple exercise, which will demonstrate to you the effects of not relaxing. Sit in a straight-backed chair. Stretch out both arms in front of you and clench your fists, or hold onto the arms of the chair very tightly. Time yourself for 60 seconds, calling out 15-second intervals. By the end of the 60 seconds, you'll feel extremely uncomfortable. Your muscles will ache and you'll be perspiring. Imagine hours of clenching yourself into a fist and you'll know how important it is to learn to relax.

There's something else rather important that you must remember about tension and relaxation. Often you won't realize that you are responding to pain by tensing up. Much of your response will be unconscious. That's why it's important to recondition your body to respond automatically by practicing simulated contractions and relaxing. It's also why your coach has to learn to recognize signs of tension and to learn to give you the signals that will enable your new conditioning to take over.

Keep in mind that relaxation is one of the most important things you'll learn. It isn't easy to learn to relax, but it must be practiced and, above all, taken seriously, even if you feel as if you're being asked to relax during the least relaxing event of your life!

Memo to the Coach

You are one of the keys to the success of this technique; your role is extremely important. You give the cues that bring the techniques into play; you are the source of support and encouragement. Through the first, sometimes long hours of labor, you'll be the only person who will share the experience with the woman in labor. So pay attention to these lessons and learn along with her. Because in the end, she's not the only one having the baby: you both are.

Remember that you will be learning to relax in a quiet, pleasant environment but you will eventually be expected to relax in a labor room of a hospital, with nurses and doctors scurrying about, doing things to you while you are experiencing the pain of labor. Practice hard. Learn relaxation so well that it will become second nature. Once you've conditioned yourself properly, you'll be able to call upon your skills in other stress- and pain-related situations.

One reason you can get through the pain of childbirth and can cope with your pain is simply that, as we have mentioned, childbirth is finite. The pain ends. You don't look back, ideally, and you don't look ahead. (Someone in one of our classes once asked how many contractions there are in the average labor. We answered, "If we told you, say, 10,622, would you ever go through with this? What are you going to do—count?")

To learn to relax, start by practicing *not* relaxing. Lie down in a comfortable position or sit in a soft, pillowy chair and try to tense each part of your body, individually, then relax it. Tense your arm. Relax it. Do you feel the difference? If you do, then you'll know what you're aiming for. If not, here's what you can do to help.

Think of the place you feel most relaxed. Is it in a hot bath, with soap bubbles floating about, soft music on your cassette player, a glass of wine on the edge of the tub? Is it sitting in front of a crackling fire after a day skiing, sipping an Irish coffee, curled up in your favorite someone's arms? It has to be a situation in which you feel calm. Describe your feelings to yourself, then write them down into a short paragraph. Here, for instance, is a sample exposition on the calm of a Caribbean island:

> You're lying on the beach. The waves are lapping at your toes. You've just had two piña coladas, and you feel pleasantly drowsy. The sun is hot as it beats down, but a cool breeze fans you gently so you're hardly aware of the heat. You're getting very sleepy now, and you think you might just drift off with the sound of the ocean a distant buzz in your ears.

Doesn't that sound nice? If you don't want to write your own and you happen to like Caribbean islands, use this example. Have your coach read it out loud to you as you lie in a comfortable position. His or her voice should be slow, soothing, even monotonous, with very little inflection. Have the coach stretch out the syllables and repeat the paragraph several times, four or five at least. Feel your body relax, close your eyes and drift. This is relaxation. This is how you should be able to make yourself feel on command.

To learn how to reach this state quickly, you must practice exercises with your coach. You can take turns, switching places regularly, so that your coach too understands the difference between relaxed and unrelaxed. One of you takes a comfortable position on the floor, on a bed or couch; the other kneels close by. The person lying down must tense each part of his or her body. Then the coach will reach out and stroke that part, telling the tense person to relax in a soft, quiet voice.

Memo to the Coach

The touch used for stroking should be light and gentle, but not so light as to be ticklish; it should be firm but not harsh. Remember that your job is not to distract her but to soothe her. And keep in mind that your tone of voice as you stroke will make all the difference to your partner; keep it soothing, even, well modulated, and caring.

Do every single part of the body, starting at the top with the head and neck, and moving all the way down to the toes. Do each side one at a time. Then switch positions with your partner. As the coach strokes, be aware of the tension and let the muscle relax in response to the touch. Eventually no words are necessary and a simple stroking will suffice. You'll learn to relax automatically in response.

Vary this exercise with one in which the coach calls out specific parts of the body. "Tense your right leg," the coach says. The woman then tenses it. He strokes. She relaxes. This helps to increase your awareness of the major muscles in your body and makes you realize the possibility of your being tense in all parts of your body. As a final exercise at the end of the session, have the person lying down tense a muscle but not say which one. The person acting as coach has to find it, stroke it, and relieve the tension. Practice the exercises lying on your side or sitting up. Do these exercises every night, without fail. They're nice to do just before you go to sleep.

The state of relaxation you aim for should be complete: loose, limp, heavy limbs. Be extra aware of certain problem areas that are sources of stress during labor. One is the jaw, which is key because it probably means that you are tensing your shoulders, face, and neck as well. The other is the perineum, the area between the vagina and anus, and tension here also means tense thighs, stomach, and buttocks. Learning to relax the perineum is especially important preparation for labor and delivery; you must relax your perineum while you are pushing just before the baby is delivered. The Kegel exercises, described in the next chapter, will help you learn how to relax the perineum.

You and your coach should aim for a totally nonverbal approach to relaxation, so that shouting "Relax, dammit!" will not be necessary. If the coach does want to speak, then make sure it's in a slow, gentle voice. He should be aware of how a muscle feels when it's relaxed so that simply by touching any part of the body he'll know if that muscle is being tensed or not.

By learning to communicate through touch, by increasing your body awareness, by sharpening your understanding of the difference between tension and relaxation, you are developing skills that will help you not only with relaxing but with applying these principles to the next most important area of instruction, the principles of breathing. Relaxation will become a part of the breathing exercises that you will learn for each phase of your labor.

CHAPTER SEVEN

Let's Get Physical: Exercises for Childbirth

Now that you've learned the basic principles and mastered relaxation techniques, it's time to turn to the first part of your reconditioning—the physical. It's extremely important to follow some regimen of physical conditioning throughout your pregnancy, but do not undertake anything—not these exercises or any other program of exercise or athletics—without speaking to your doctor first. We repeat: do not attempt the exercises in this book unless you have your doctor's permission.

Physical conditioning is vital because labor and delivery are, above all, physical events. You must prepare your body to be flexible, because you will assume positions during this time that may be difficult to get into, particularly when you're carrying all that extra baby weight and bulk. Labor nurses know this quite well; we've seen 250-pound women who've never exercised and who are so out of shape they cannot even lift their legs up so their babies can be delivered. In addition to simple flexibility, exercise will improve your stamina, your breathing, your posture, and your muscle tone during the time you carry the baby prior to delivery. Your circulation will be improved as well.

With your doctor's permission, you can exercise throughout your entire pregnancy. Here are some very simple exercises. If you do them every day, they will help you enormously. If you are already engaged in a physical program of your own, you can use these exercises to supplement what you already do. They are designed to help you specifically with the physical demands of childbirth. It would be even better if this program were supplemented by additional regular exercise, but if you're already well advanced into your pregnancy, then doing only these exercises will help.

Before you attempt these exercises, keep these things in mind: never do them after you have eaten (if you've eaten a heavy meal, wait several hours), when you're tired, or when your legs ache. And *remember:* talk to your doctor first! You'll notice that there's a lot of emphasis on legs and hips; this is because when you're pushing during the end of labor, you'll need all the strength you can get in order to assist in delivering the baby. Strength in this area is always appreciated for that last, long haul.

Follow these simple rules for all exercises:

1. Keep your pelvis stable. Don't shift your body from side to side.

2. Never compress your abdomen. That is, don't bend over your stomach and press down on the baby.
3. Do not exaggerate any of the movements.
4. Do not point your toes. You'll get leg cramps.
5. When you must lie down or stand up, get up and down from the side. Don't stand up from a flat position or try to lie down directly onto your back.
6. Wear something loose-fitting or flexible.
7. Do the exercises at the same time each day. This will help you remember to keep the exercise habit.
8. Lie on a carpet or exercise mat.
9. If anything starts to hurt, stop immediately!

The Tailor Reach

The first exercise is a simple warm-up, stretching exercise (*see Figures 2 and 3*). Sit on the floor with your legs crossed Indian-style (the tailor sit). This exercise will improve the tone of the upper part of your body, your pectorals, and your spinal muscles, as well as improve ventilation. You are going to coordinate breathing with your arm movement. Take a deep, cleansing breath, in through the nose and out through the mouth, and begin. With your right hand, reach toward the ceiling as you inhale. Breath in as you reach, stretching up as if you were grabbing for thousand-dollar bills dangling just out of your grasp. Your left arm is at your side, your hand resting on your knee. Hold this stretch as long as you can without straining, then begin to lower your arm slowly, exhaling as you do so. Then repeat with your left arm, leaving your right arm at your side, hand resting on your knee. Do this five times to begin with, slowly increasing every day as much as you like. A maximum of twenty times, ten for each side, might be a good goal.

The Tailor Reach

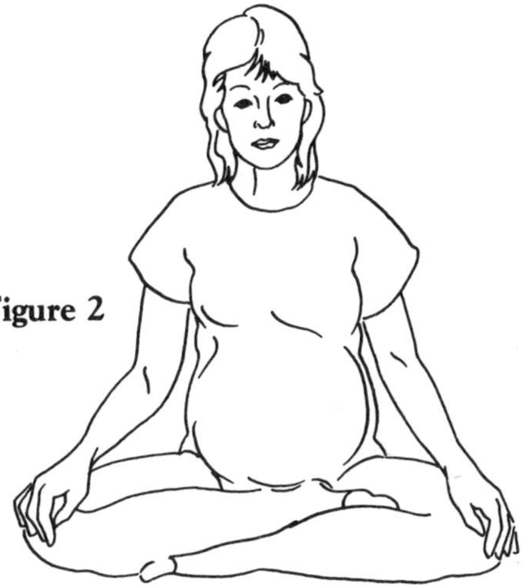

Figure 2

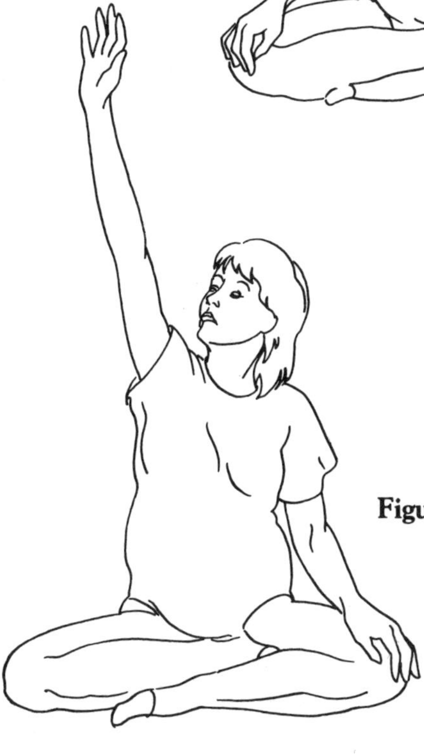

Figure 3

The Tailor Press

For the next exercise (*see Figures 4, 5, and 6*), you remain seated on the floor, but instead of crossing your legs, stretch out your calves and press the soles of your feet together. Don't bring your legs in too close to your body: just sit comfortably, without straining. To warm up for this exercise, which is going to increase flexibility in the hip and leg area as well as relieve tension and lower-back distress, simply bounce your knees for thirty seconds to loosen your leg muscles. Now, with your back straight, take a deep, cleansing breath, in through the nose and out through the mouth, and begin. Inhale, and lift your knees toward the ceiling. You'll feel a stretching in your thighs. As you inhale, lift your knees up very slowly. Then as you start to exhale, press your knees toward the floor; do this movement gradually, so that you do not feel too much strain. This exercise should be done very slowly. Your hands and arms are not involved and may be kept in a relaxed position. Again, this may be done five times to start, slowly increasing the number each day until you work up to ten times. With this and all the exercises, remember to breathe and to coordinate your breathing with the exercising as indicated. That is extremely important. You're not working your muscles properly unless you do your breathing.

The Tailor Press

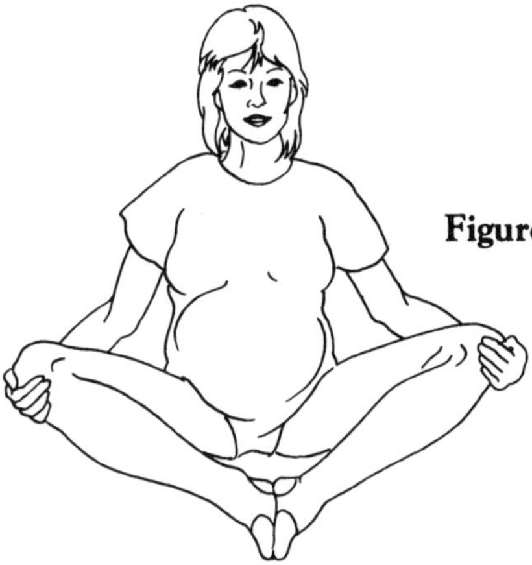

Figure 4

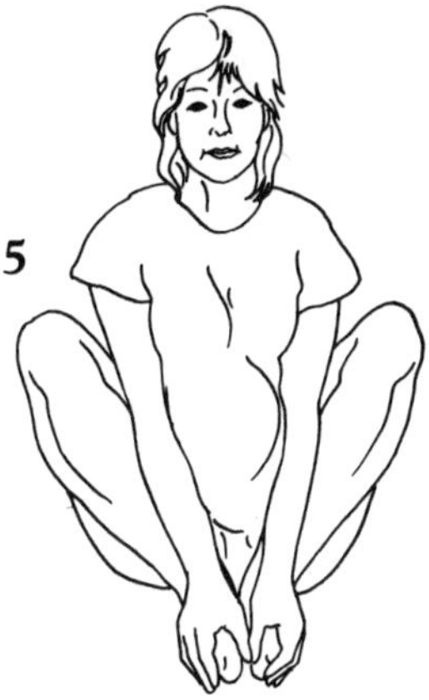

Figure 5

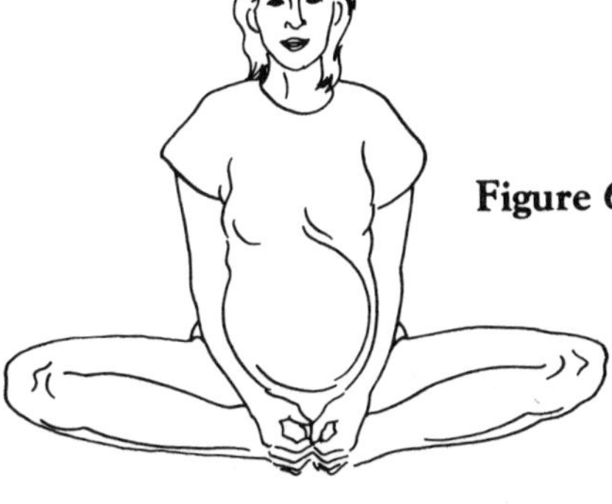

Figure 6

The Tailor Stretch

Stay seated on the floor for the next exercise (*see Figures 7 and* 8). Spread your legs, but not too far; don't strain. Allow your feet to remain flexed. (Remember, if you point your toes, you'll get leg cramps.) During this exercise, it's essential not to bend over too far, curling your body, as you will compress your abdomen right on top of your baby. Again, take a cleansing breath and begin the exercise. Keeping your outstretched arms parallel to your leg, bend first to the right, to a count of three, stretching toward your foot, then straighten up and repeat to the left side. Your breathing should be coordinated so that you inhale before you stretch and exhale on the stretch. Sit up between bendings and inhale before you move to the other side. Start with five times to each side and work up to ten times for each side. Remember to keep your body at a 90 degree angle; never bend over more than that. This is good for both your hip and leg muscles as well as your lower back and waist.

The Tailor Stretch

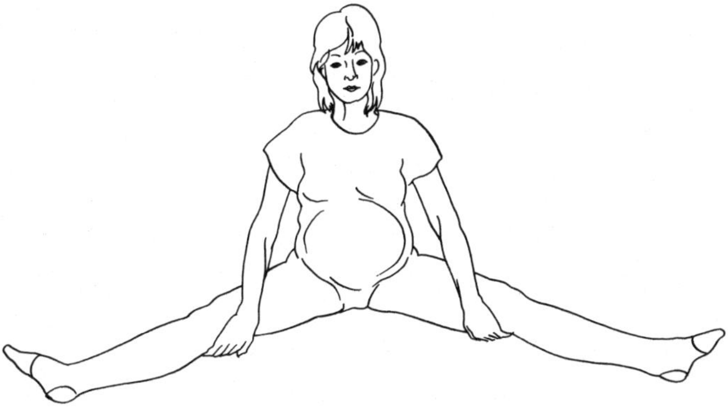

Figure 7

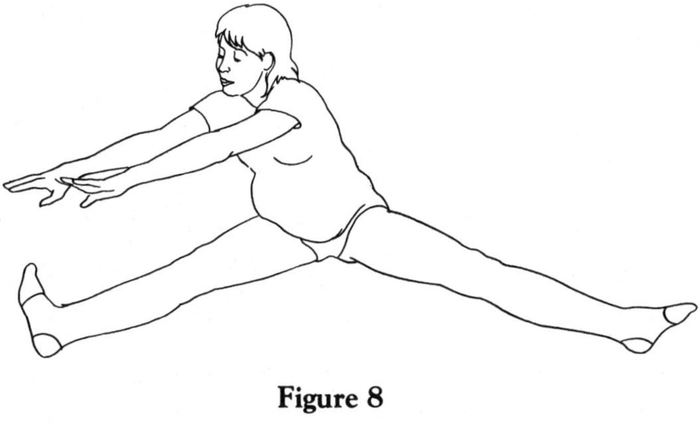

Figure 8

The Pelvic Tilt

This is one of the most important of all the exercises, though it may seem relatively simple. It is important to make certain you are doing it correctly, so have your husband or coach nearby to help the first time you try it. This exercise (*see Figures 9 and 10*) is excellent for abdominal muscle tone, and it is marvelous if you're having backaches. Lie flat on the floor, knees bent, hands outstretched at your sides. Have the person assisting you kneel down alongside you and place his or her hand under the small of your back. You will then slowly roll your waist toward the floor, as you exhale. Your buttocks should remain on the floor, though they may lift slightly as you do the exercise. Roll your spine from your buttocks toward your neck, so that your back touches the floor as it curves. The person with you will feel your spine touch the hand beneath you; that is how you can tell you're doing the exercise correctly. Curve your spine back up so you're lying normally, as you were when you began, and as you do so, inhale. You will always be exhaling on the roll toward the floor. Do this exercise five times to begin with and work your way up to as many as you like. It's not a strenuous exercise, but it yields excellent results and, in the process, can be very relaxing if you do it in an unhurried fashion, taking slow breaths.

The Pelvic Tilt

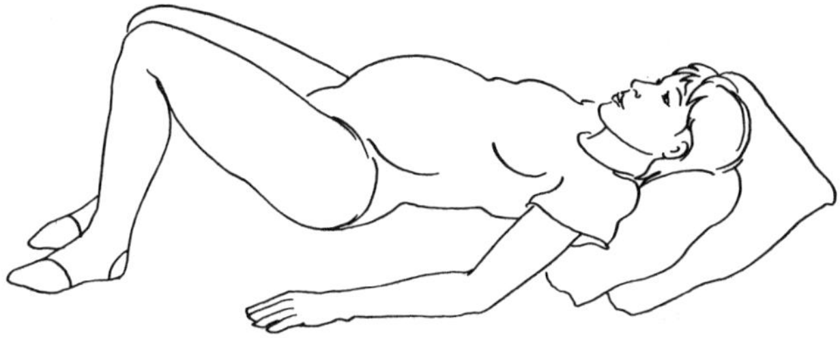

Figure 9

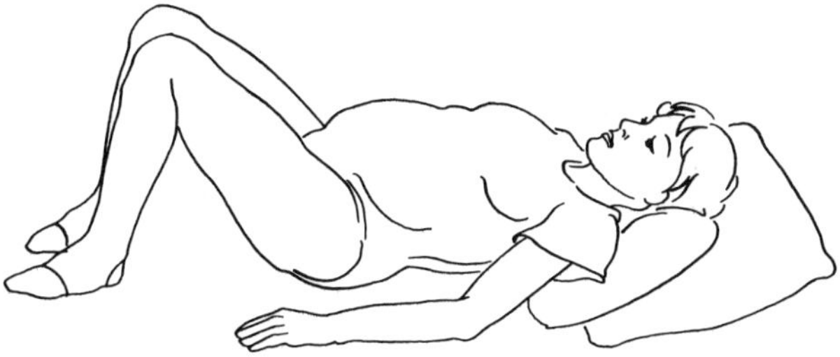

Figure 10

The Bent Leg Lift

Stay on your back for this one, which will increase muscle flexibility in your legs and hips as well as improve circulation in your lower body. (*See Figures 11, 12, 13, and 14.*) Bend both legs. Begin with the right leg, and as you do the exercise, be careful not to rock from side to side. Keep your pelvis stable as you do it. You will lift the right leg, with the knee bent, toward your head to the count of one, then at two, extend the leg slowly, and three to four, slowly lower the leg so that it ends up stretched out on the floor. Return your leg to its bent-knee position and switch to the left leg. Inhale as you raise the leg toward you, slowly, then exhale very slowly as you stretch the leg out and lower it. Start with five times per leg and work up to ten times for each leg.

The Bent Leg Lift

Figure 11

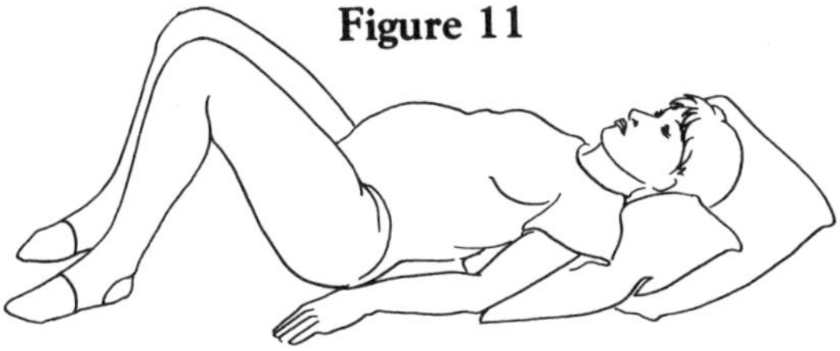

Figure 12

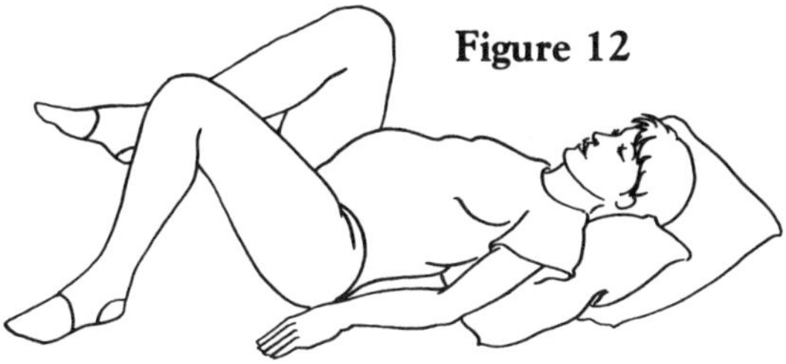

Figure 13

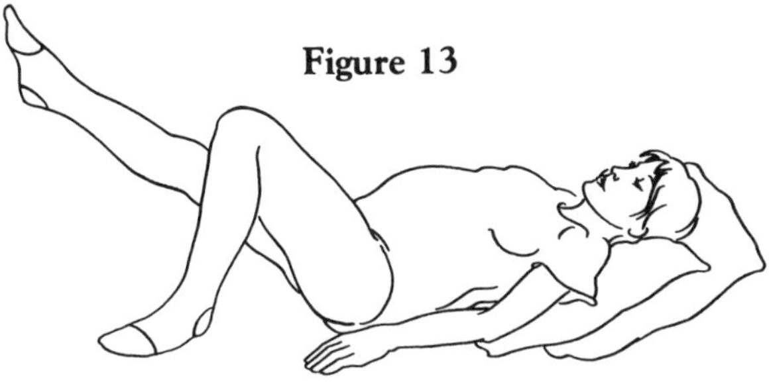

Figure 14

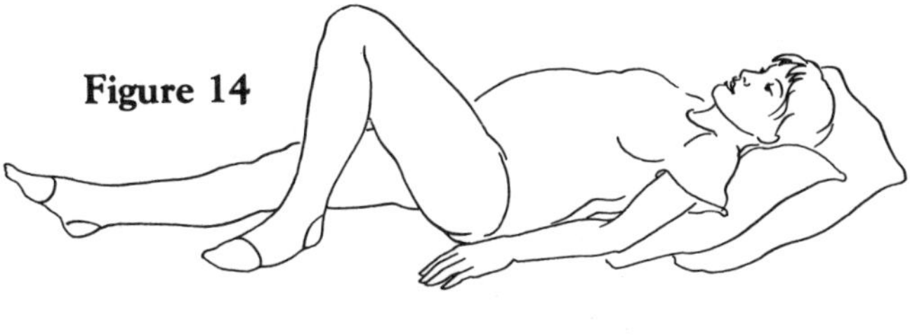

The Back Roll

This is a crucial exercise for the second stage of labor, during which your body will be required to assume a similar position. (*See Figures 15, 16, and 17.*) Stay flat on the floor, again, and remember, too, in this exercise not to make more than a 90 degree angle with your body. Don't compress your abdomen. Your legs and back will benefit a great deal from this simple exercise. Bend your knees before you start. On the count of one, inhale and raise both legs, still bent, toward your head. On two, raise your head and shoulders off the ground, exhale, and move them toward your legs. Remember to keep the angle gentle: don't force this movement. As you finish exhaling, both your legs and shoulders should be raised. On three, inhale, and slowly let your head and shoulders down. On four, exhale, and let your legs down again. Your breathing and your movements should be slow. This exercise may not seem to do much, but it does simulate a position you will assume in labor, and it will help build up your endurance. Begin with five times and work up to ten.

The Back Roll

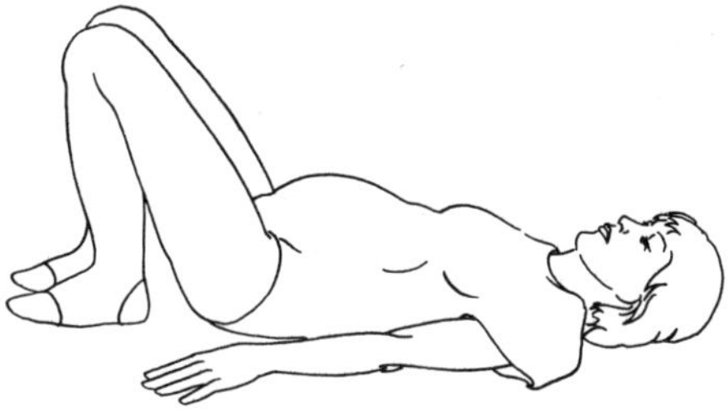

Figure 15

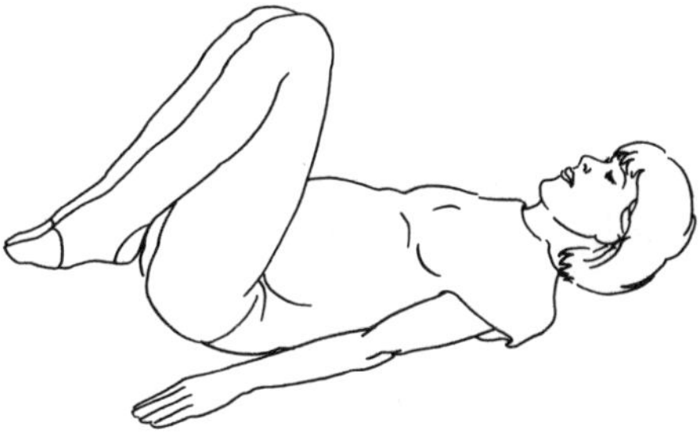

Figure 16

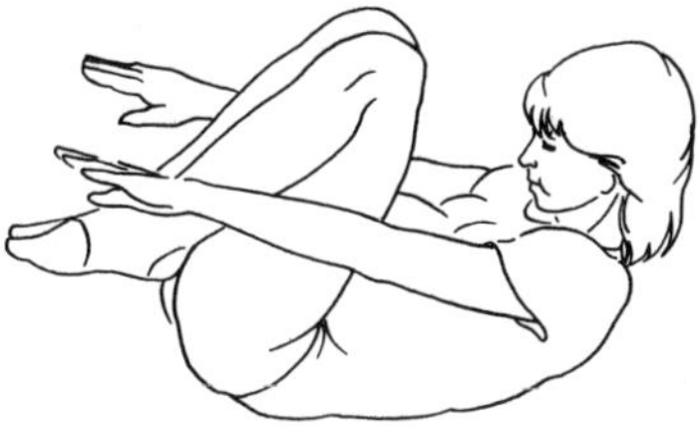

Figure 17

Kegels

Last, but by no means least, is a subtle little exercise known as the Kegel. Kegels can be done anywhere: in the subway, in the office, in front of the television, in the shower. In fact, Kegels *should* be done everywhere. The more Kegels you do, the better it is for your muscle tone in your vagina. It's easy to do a Kegel; simply contract your vaginal muscles. You're not sure how? Pretend you're urinating and you want to stop the flow, just for an instant. Feel it? If you're not sure, try pretending you've got a tampon inside that's threatening to slip out. If all else fails and you can't get the hang of this exercise, try it on your husband. He'll tell you if you're contracting or not.

Do all these exercises as often as possible. If you do, you'll be able to keep yourself flexible enough to have an easier time during labor and delivery.

CHAPTER EIGHT

Whatever Gets You Through the Night: The Art of Breathing

Relaxation and exercise play important parts in childbirth, but the key part of your prepared childbirth experience is breathing. Breathing is what will get you through the night. Combined with your relaxation techniques, it can be an effective tool in reducing the pain and tension of labor and in enabling the mother, should she choose, to have a delivery free of any interference, provided there are no complications.

How does something as simple as breathing work to help make your labor better? There are two main reasons. The first is physiological. The uterus is a muscle, and when a muscle contracts—as the uterus does in labor—the oxygen supply is cut down markedly. The muscle is oxygen-starved, and it hurts. But inside the uterus is a baby, who is also greatly in need of oxygen. When you're in pain, it's common to hold your breath as you tense, waiting for the pain to pass. If you hold your breath during all the contractions that make up a normal labor, you're making it far more difficult for your oxygen-deprived uterus and for the baby as well. This isn't life-threatening, but your labor will be tougher. Like proper breathing during exercise, breathing correctly during labor helps the body to get rid of the waste products produced by the working muscles. The results are less pain and more energy.

The second reason is psychological. Breathing during labor is a special kind of breathing: it's rhythmic; it has to be learned very carefully; it requires concentration; and in spite of what you may think, it is not "natural." Many of the techniques described here are exactly what we don't do when we breathe normally. This difficulty provides a great distraction from the actual contractions. If you do your rhythmic breathing exercises in a certain, patterned way in response to a contraction, the sixty seconds of that contraction will go a great deal faster than if you held your breath for sixty seconds. You are, quite simply, thinking of something other than the pain.

In addition, patterned breathing is designed to work in conjunction with the natural response of your body to labor: as the contractions get more difficult, part of the body's response is to increase the pulse rate, increase the blood pressure, increase the respiratory rate. In order to accommodate this natural flow, the patterned breathing increases its rate in the progression as the contractions get stronger. Since this is what your body wants to do, it makes the breathing pattern seem even more natural.

And, of course, the stronger the contraction, the more complicated the breathing pattern called upon in response. Thus you have to concentrate that much harder, and you are that much more distracted from the pain. The breathing is more difficult as the labor gets more difficult; the breathing gets faster as the labor gets harder.

Before we explain the breathing techniques, we want to remind you once more of the four fundamentals of technique that were discussed in Chapter 5, since these are especially important to your breathing exercises. These techniques will help to decrease stress, increase concentration, and decrease the amount of distraction.

1. Always get into a *comfortable position.*
2. Choose a *focal point* and concentrate on it during all your exercises.
3. Use your *verbal and nonverbal cues* and keep them in mind.
4. Don't forget that *deep, cleansing breath* at the beginning and the end of each contraction.

Memo to the Coach

In order to help you both to remember these fundamentals, each time you practice a contraction, tell her, "Okay, find a comfortable position, get your focal point, take a deep breath in and out." If you say that every time, soon it will be second nature to you both.

Pregnant women customarily learn breathing at twenty-eight to thirty weeks, near the time of delivery, but with some time to spare to practice. There are two basic breathing techniques that you must learn first. You must practice these two techniques separately for at least *one week* before you move on to any other breathing exercises. Remember, a week's practice of each of these two comes first.

Figure 18: Slow Chest Breathing

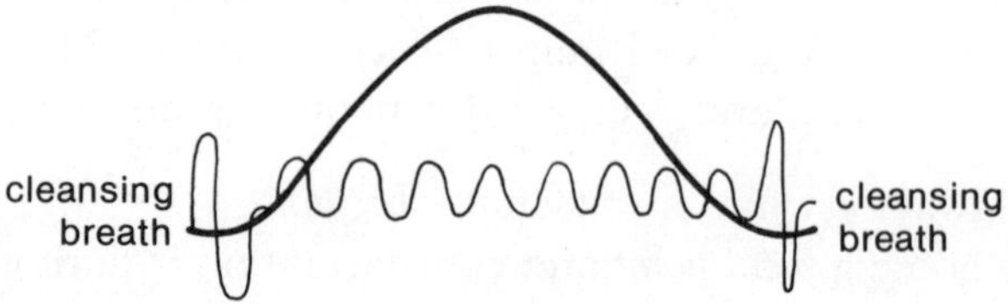

Slow Chest Breathing

Number one, slow chest breathing, is slow and rhythmic, with the air taken deeply into the chest. (*See Figure 18.*) It is more strongly connected to the diaphragm than to the lungs, though when you are pregnant you may find it more difficult than usual to make this distinction, since the baby's bulk compresses your midsection. You inhale deeply through your nose and exhale through a relaxed mouth. When you first try this breathing, use a simple counting method, to slow beats, to time how deep your breaths are: inhale . . . two . . . three . . . four, exhale . . . two . . . three . . . four. Your mouth, when you exhale, should remain open only slightly, very relaxed and loose. Don't tense up your face, please. Check in a mirror or ask your coach if you are grimacing or not. You should, when you inhale, be able to feel the air go deeply into your lungs, but this breathing should not be as exaggerated as your cleansing breaths. Just keep the breathing very even and very full. Think of a film running in slow motion.

Practice this breathing in the following manner: keep your fundamentals of technique firmly in mind; practice the slow chest breathing eight times per minute; stop and wait a few minutes between each practice contraction, then repeat. Practice this breathing five times per day or night. Try to shut out all stimuli by concentrating on your focal point, and, between practice minutes, practice relaxing.

Figure 19: Shallow Chest Breathing

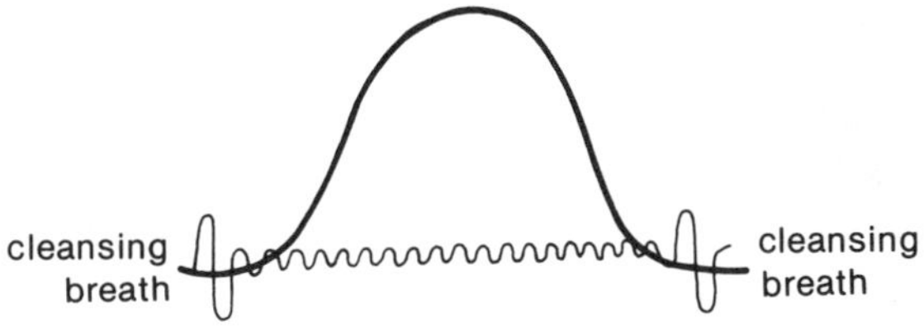

Shallow Chest Breathing

The next technique, shallow chest breathing, is not as deep as slow chest. You are going to bring the air only halfway into your chest, and you may feel this breathing more in the chest and lungs than in the diaphragm. (*See Figure 19.*) This is also a faster breathing. You inhale through your mouth and exhale through your mouth. Your mouth should be open gently, very loose and relaxed. The breathing is light, effortless, and shallow, with a slight emphasis on exhalation. It is as if you were making an "H" sound without speaking. To understand the difference between the two breathing techniques, put your hands on your chest and compare the deep and shallow breathing. With shallow breathing, you are more aware of your chest rising and falling.

Practice this breathing, again keeping the fundamentals of technique in mind, 60 times per minute or 1 breath every second. If this breathing is not done properly—that is, if you breathe in too deeply while trying to breathe this fast—you may begin to hyperventilate, which means you are blowing off too much carbon dioxide. You'll begin to feel dizzy, lightheaded, and tingly in the fingertips and lips. If this happens to you, cup your hands over your nose and mouth and breathe deeply and normally into your hands for several minutes until you feel better. Hyperventilating isn't very dangerous but you should avoid doing it. Then, when you next practice shallow chest breathing, don't take the air in so far. If you are having problems with doing this breathing properly, try making an "S" or hissing sound when you exhale in order to help you get the right emphasis. Do this breathing five times per day in addition to the slow chest breathing.

When you start, you may feel exhausted and out of breath, and your mouth may feel dry. This is not unusual. Shallow breathing is not natural, and your diaphragm is being pushed up inside your body by the growing body of your baby. At the beginning, you may feel unable to do any of it, but keep practicing, because the more you try it, the easier it will be and, eventually, it will be close to second nature. Set aside a particular time every day and do your breathing. Remember, five times for each kind of breathing, and separate each practice minute by at least several minutes of relaxation in between. Do this for at least a week before moving on.

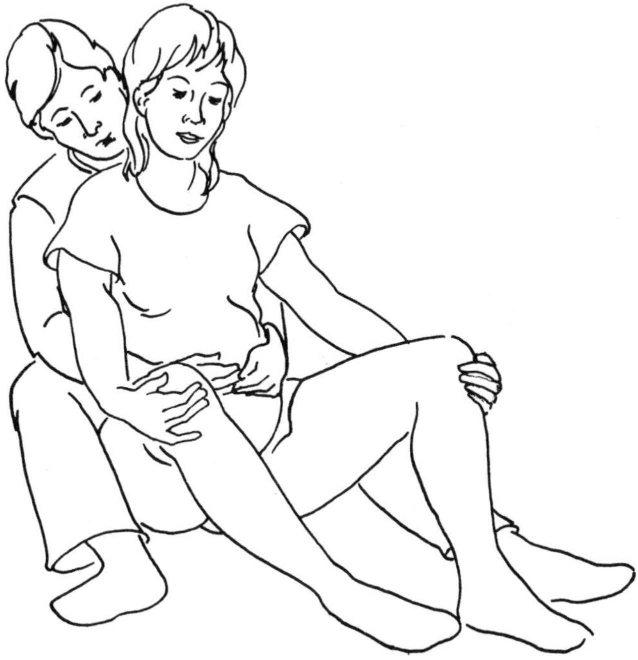

Figure 20: You may want to lean up against your partner or a friend so that you can breathe through contractions together.

Memo to the Coach

Learn to do the breathing along with her. You should become as accomplished at these breathing techniques as she is. This is the only way you'll be able to understand what she's doing. You will be responsible for telling her whether she's doing her breathing correctly or not, so get down there on the floor, lie on your side, and breathe!

The progression of breathing, which is the combination of techniques that will get you through labor, is very systematic. Each type of breathing follows in sequence. It starts with the easy forms of breathing and progresses to the more difficult, just as labor itself does. What you must remember is that you are to do these breathing techniques at your own level according to your own ability. You set your own pace during your labor. You will move on, from one technique to another, only when the breathing you have been doing previously no longer holds you through a contraction. You will know when this happens or your coach will; your breathing will be more labored and will be harder to do. Your breathing may be too slow for the stronger contractions and you may be speeding up unnecessarily. But *there is no set time* to change. There are six techniques in this breathing progression. Use them as you need them in your labor but do what gets you through, not what you think you're supposed to be doing. You're allowed to be flexible.

Breathing Progression

Figure 21: Slow Chest Breathing

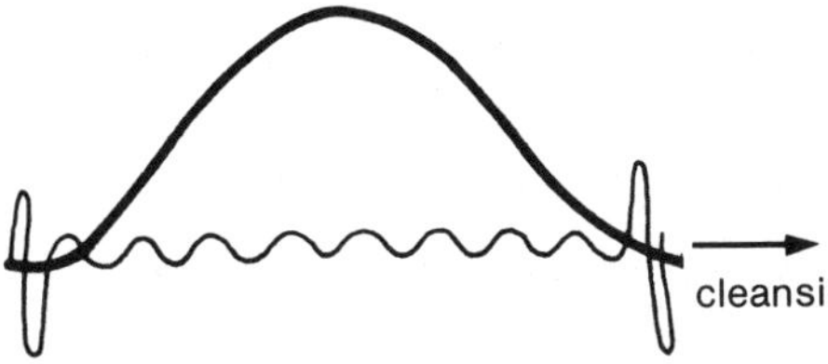

*1. **Slow Chest Breathing.*** You've just learned this kind of breathing: in through the nose and out through the mouth, 8 times per minute. This is customarily used in the early stages of labor. It's a comfortable kind of breathing, very relaxed, and helpful when the contractions are not very strong.

Figure 22: Modified Slow Chest Breathing

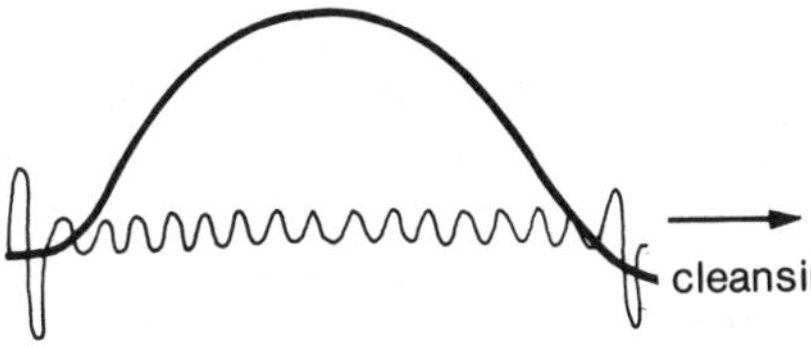

*2. **Modified Slow Chest Breathing.*** This is slow chest breathing done at double the rate you've been practicing, 16 times per minute, which is approximately the rate of normal breathing. It will come automatically in the progression; as your labor gets a bit stronger, you'll want to speed up naturally and you will. No one will have to signal this change to you; it will simply happen.

Figure 23: Combined Pattern

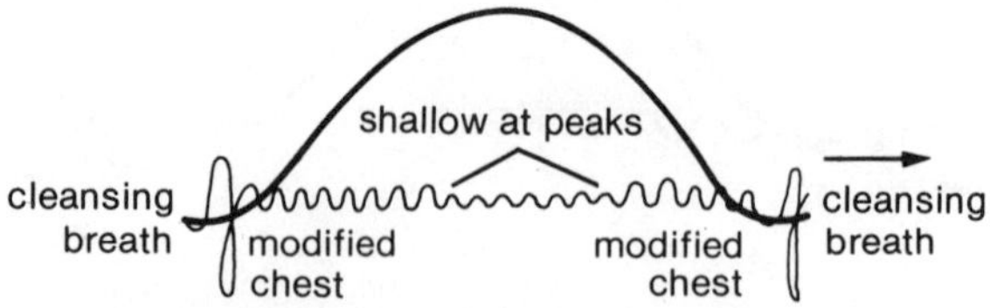

3. Combined Pattern. After a while, the contractions you've been having begin to peak earlier: contractions are like mountain climbing, an ascent up a hill to a peak, then a gradual decline down. Earlier in labor this peaking is not very noticeable, but as your labor advances, the middle will be stronger than the beginning or the end of the contraction. You'll want to use a type of breathing that will help you in the middle without exhausting you at the beginning or the end. The combined pattern is modified slow chest breathing at a rate of 16 per minute at the beginning and at the end, with a shift in the middle to shallow chest breathing. Practice this as follows, remembering always, as with all forms of breathing, to take a deep, cleansing breath at the beginning and at the end. Have your coach help you with dividing up your minute of practice time into 15-second intervals. After the first 15 seconds, the contraction begins to peak, so you switch from your modified slow chest breathing to shallow chest breathing. From 15 to 45 seconds, you'll do the shallow chest breathing, in through the mouth and out through the mouth. Then at 45 seconds you'll switch back to modified slow chest breathing.

Here is where the coach will begin to get some practice telling you when to switch to a different breathing technique. He can say "switch" or whatever the two of you determine might help you to remember to make the change. When you're in labor, he won't need to consult a watch; he'll be able to tell from looking at your face and listening to your breathing that it's time to switch. You'll be grimacing and breathing in a labored fashion. Remember that the shallow chest breathing is the most tiring of all the kinds of breathing, and when you're in labor you only want to do it when it's absolutely necessary. If the modified chest breathing is getting you through, by all means stick with it. There's no reason to change unless you absolutely have to.

Figure 24: Shallow Accelerated-Decelerated Chest Breathing

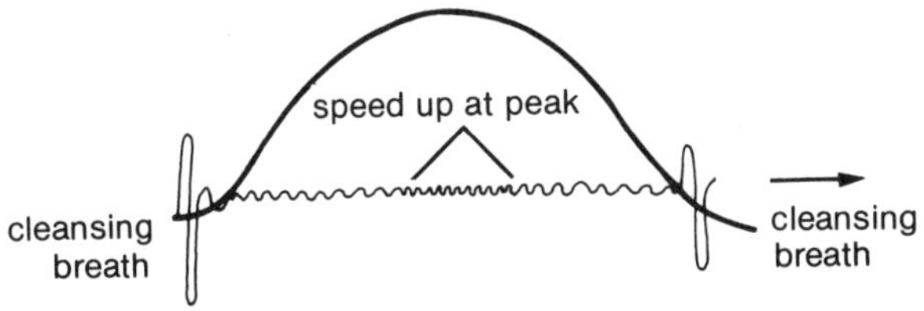

4. Shallow Accelerated-Decelerated Chest Breathing. This is usually employed during active labor, when the contractions are much stronger and the peaks are coming very quickly. By this time, the beginning and the end of the contractions may not be much of a bargain, either. To get through a more difficult beginning and on to a strong middle, you may begin with shallow chest breathing done at a slower rate of 60 per minute, gradually accelerating speed as you reach the peak, and as the contraction gets better, slowing down gradually until the contraction is over. Start as slowly as you can, around 60 breaths per minute, and work your way up to about 120 per minute. The slower you start, the more you can speed up as you need to. Give yourself some leeway. This should be a gentle acceleration and deceleration; work your way up and down at a moderate rate. No greatly exaggerated switches from one speed to another, please. That could leave you exhausted and lightheaded. And with the use of only shallow breathing, you will discover that your mouth will become uncomfortably dry. (In Chapter 11, you'll be instructed as to what to pack in your prepared childbirth bag; you'll have lip balm for dry lips and sour lollipops to increase the flow of saliva. The hospital will also give you ice chips to suck on.)

Figure 25: Rhythmic Pattern

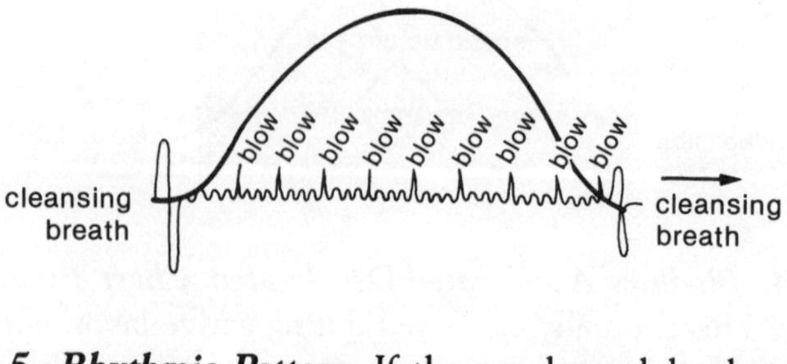

5. Rhythmic Pattern. If the accelerated-decelerated method is not working as well as it might as your labor becomes more intense, you can use the rhythmic pattern, which has the advantage of providing you with some variation in breathing that can prove more helpful during the difficult moments. This consists of three shallow breaths, with every third breath followed by a gentle blow—not as exaggerated as one required to blow out a match but a definite puff of air. Remember to take three complete shallow breaths, inhale and then blow. The sequence is as follows: inhale/exhale, inhale/exhale, inhale/exhale, inhale/*blow*. This can be accelerated and decelerated as necessary, starting off slowly and gradually getting faster at the peak of the contractions.

Figure 26: Advanced Rhythmic Pattern

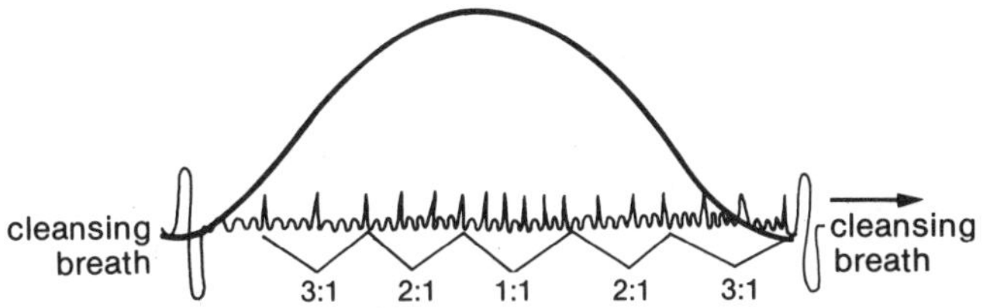

6. Advanced Rhythmic Pattern. Toward the end of labor, you'll want to use some of these more complicated patterns as they require a lot of thought and will be very distracting, as well as providing the necessary increased oxygen the baby will need for the last and hardest part of the birth. Start off using three shallow breaths and one blow, as described in the method above, the rhythmic pattern. Vary this with two breaths and one blow as the contraction gets stronger, and as it peaks, use one breath and one blow. As the contraction begins to decline in intensity, switch back to two breaths, one blow, then to three breaths, one blow. This is the most complicated breathing pattern of all and the one that requires the most concentrated practice. Separate the contraction into 15-second intervals, lengthening the time period you use to a minute and 15 seconds. For the first 15 seconds, use three breaths and one blow; from 15 to 30 seconds, use two breaths and one blow; 30–45 seconds, one breath and one blow; 45–60 seconds, two breaths and one blow; 60–75 seconds, three breaths and one blow. Learn this pattern slowly; don't rush through the practice sessions. If you learn it slowly, you can always speed it up. For the first few practice sessions, it might even be a good idea if you tried the breathing without timing until you have mastered the switching back and forth with ease.

This is an opportunity for the coach to practice using hand signals with the woman so that she becomes accustomed to some nonverbal cues. During labor, she may not want to hear someone calling out "switch," and so by simply practicing holding up one, two, or three fingers, you can coordinate your timing in advance. And in labor, the coach will be able to tell by watching the woman's face whether it's time for her to switch to another kind of breathing. Blowing, especially in the one-and-one relationship at the peak of the contraction, also helps prevent you from pushing, which is a very strong urge at the end of labor but which you must not do until you're given the okay by your doctor or midwife. The blowing will help curb that urge.

The most important thing to remember about practicing these six forms of breathing is to *practice them from number 1 to number* 6, *in order.* Your labor will also progress, just as the breathing does, from the simplest of contractions to the hardest work, so advance your breathing accordingly. When you are in actual labor, some of the contractions may seem worse than others, so if one comes along that isn't so bad, don't be afraid to go back to an easier form of breathing. But *don't skip ahead.* Don't bypass the next stage of breathing and move to the most complicated. Always try the next method. If you don't and you move ahead too quickly, when your labor gets really tough you'll feel as if you have nothing to fall back on. So always try the next stage of breathing. Learn the progression in order and use it in order. When you switch breathing, and which breathing you use for which stage, is entirely up to you. Some women have delivered babies using only slow chest breathing the entire way through. Some women are happier with one of the combinations. Be flexible. And let your coach help you remember your order and the progression. This is where the coach becomes invaluable.

Memo to the Coach

When you have mastered, together, the six breathing methods, you can add to your practice technique to improve your performance. For instance, when you've become accustomed to the 15-second intervals, try not to consult your watch or a clock for each interval. A problem many coaches have is that sometimes they spend more time looking at their watches than at their wives. It's more important for you to make sure her arms, legs, jaw, and shoulders are relaxed during the contractions, so start getting used to using approximate times to tell her it's peaking or it's nearly over.

The method to use with your coach when practicing is as follows:

1. Have the coach do all the breathing along with you. Practice each type of breathing, using the fundamentals of technique for each and every one. Go through all six types, at least two times, together. You may be in labor for quite a while at home, and the coach must supervise breathing. In the hospital, there are many times when you'll be alone with your coach, so let your coach learn as you learn.

2. Next, have your coach watch you go through the breathing progression. Do all six, employing the fundamentals of technique, and repeat the whole thing twice.

3. Do the breathing and let the coach begin his job of helping you. He should be employing techniques of relaxation, stroking, using verbal cues, encouraging you. Again, go through all six twice.

Effleurage and Pressure

When the breathing has become second nature, you can add the technique known as effleurage. This stimulus, which you can use in conjunction with breathing and relaxation, can be practiced with the simulated contractions for the earlier stages of labor; in later stages of labor, though, it can become more distracting than it's worth. Effleurage is a series of light, gentle, circular strokes on the abdomen made by the woman with her fingertips. It's a light massage, with both hands making symmetrical circles on the abdomen. Each hand makes its circle toward the other: one hand moves clockwise, the other counterclockwise. It can feel very good during labor, and it serves as a reminder to relax. It is important to remember not to do effleurage at the same rate as your breathing, which is why you should learn and practice the breathing first. Add the effleurage later and keep it at the same slow, steady rhythm regardless of how quickly your breathing may be. Wildly circling your abdomen with your hands will not help you to relax. Some women like this technique, but others do not. Practice effleurage with your breathing, and when you're in labor you can decide for yourself whether it's helpful. The coach can perform the effleurage, too, but during actual labor many women prefer not to be touched on their abdomens.

Something else you can add to your practice sessions—again, after you have mastered the breathing techniques—is pressure to simulate contractions. The coach can put his hand on your arm or leg and gradually increase the pressure during the duration of one of your practice contractions. The coach shouldn't use the fingers of the hand in a squeezing gesture, but rather the whole hand for an even application of pressure. Don't dig your fingers in! The point is not to leave bruises but to provide an uncomfortable distraction that will help the woman to understand the importance of concentration. For the more advanced breathing techniques, the coach should apply more pressure, as the contractions here will be stronger. You are going to be uncomfortable during this exercise, but try not to interrupt your concentration to yell, "Hey, that really hurts!" unless it's absolutely necessary. During labor you're not going to be able to stop your contraction in the middle. It's not easy to concentrate during labor. It takes a lot of hard work, skill, and willpower, so it's a good idea to try and see if you can develop some of this ahead of time.

Memo to the Coach

You may feel a little ridiculous calling out intervals, stroking your wife's relaxed body, grabbing her arm and applying pressure. But when labor comes, everything you have learned will be essential not only for her well-being but for yours as well. No one likes to see a loved one in pain, and what you are learning is designed to help her. Persist, practice, apply what you've learned. The payoff will come—and you won't feel silly at all.

When you have learned all the techniques of breathing, practice the sequence every day. You can limit yourself to one practice session, but go through the sequence at least twice. Do each technique for a minute, then allow a minute in between, during which you should practice your relaxation. To get through this entire sequence twice should take you no more than twenty minutes. Practice faithfully, and you'll see results. When you learn about labor in the next chapter, you'll see exactly why these techniques are called for during the different stages of labor. Everything will fit together, and you'll be prepared for the birth of your baby.

CHAPTER NINE

This Isn't Gas, This Is It—Isn't It?: The Start of Labor

You've probably heard a million stories about labor and how horrible it is. There's something about the subject that makes women want to talk about it. They relive their labors, down to the last gory detail, for anybody who asks—or doesn't ask. You may find yourself the uncomfortable listener to many tales of the delivery room, but don't believe all you hear.

Many women turn up at the labor room doors scared half to death, not by what's happening to them but by what they *think* is going to happen to them. They're afraid of pain, and this fear is compounded by the terror of the unknown. Since the best way to combat fear is with knowledge, let's start with a look at your pregnant body and at the stable situation of pregnancy.

For nine months, you've been growing a baby. Until labor begins, which is the process by which this baby is expelled from your body, the growth and nurturing of your baby involve the following things. The baby is connected to the *placenta,* an organ rich in blood vessels which nourishes the baby and also serves to excrete its waste products. The *umbilical cord,* which connects the baby from its navel to the placenta, is a long, jellylike rope containing a continuation of those blood vessels to nourish the baby. The *amniotic sac,* a membrane surrounding the baby, contains the amniotic fluid, in which the baby floats. This fluid maintains a constant temperature for the growing baby, cushions the baby against injury, provides a medium in which the baby can move, and allows for the symmetrical growth of the fetus. All of these are contained in your *uterus.* Originally a small, hollow, pear-shaped muscle located in your lower abdomen, it expands in a remarkable way as your baby grows. Then it shrinks back to its original pear size by six weeks after the baby is born. The uterus, at its bottom, ends in what is called the neck of the womb, or the *cervix,* from which the vagina extends downward. The cervix is closed and plugged with mucus during pregnancy, but when labor begins, the cervix thins out (this is called *effacement*) and then opens (this is called *dilatation*). Rhythmic contractions of the uterus will take place, and the amniotic bag may rupture as the baby's head presses down toward the opening of the cervix. The cervix will eventually open enough to admit that head, and then the body, and the baby will pass into your vagina and out to be born. The umbilical cord is cut, since it no longer serves a purpose. The placenta will be delivered following the baby; it's sometimes referred to as the *afterbirth.*

This is basically what takes place during what we call labor. Everyone's labor is different, some so unusual that the use of forceps or surgery may be necessary. These variations will be discussed in subsequent chapters. But basically everyone experiences all these stages in labor.

Before you actually go into labor, you may experience some of the things that comprise what is called the *prelude to labor*. These are not hard-and-fast events that will happen to everyone. Some people never experience any of them; others may notice just one or two. These are just small signs that your body is, indeed, readying itself to have a baby. These signs should be taken as positive hints that it's time to practice your breathing and relaxing even harder, and time to think about organizing your thoughts so that when labor does come you're not running around trying to catch up on all the little chores you've postponed.

About two to four weeks before your baby is due, one or more of the following *may* occur:

1. Lightening. This refers to the engagement of the baby's head in your pelvis. Throughout your pregnancy, the baby has been high in your body, next to your diaphragm. In the last weeks, the baby may "drop" so that its head settles down into your pelvis, in the preferred position for birth. You may notice that your breathing is easier, that you have a greater urge to urinate more frequently, and that you have become constipated. People may tell you they see a change in your shape; they'll comment that you've "dropped." The baby moves naturally into this position. Since the head is the heaviest part of the baby, gravity plays a big role. Even if this has occurred for you, however, you may not notice any change at all.

2. Increased Vaginal Discharge. In the last weeks, you may notice a whitish, creamy discharge from your vagina (not a watery leaking). It may resemble a vaginal infection, but there will be no itching or discomfort.

3. Increase of Braxton Hicks Contractions. These are irregular contractions of the uterus. They are painless, and can start as early as the fifth or sixth month of pregnancy. In the earlier months they serve no purpose; as your due date comes closer, they can increase in frequency, and you can actually feel your uterus tightening if you happen to have your hand on your belly. There may be a little effacement of the cervix taking place closer to term. For the most part the contractions are not noticeable, though at the very end they can be more regular and can be mistaken for the beginning of labor. The difference is they will not sustain; they'll remain the same in duration and not progress and eventually they'll stop.

4. Sleep Difficulties. At the end, you're carrying a lot of weight, you're uncomfortable, and you may be getting anxious, so you may have trouble sleeping. Try to relax and catch some sleep during the day if it eludes you at night.

5. Nesting Instinct. Many women have a flash of energy right at the end of their pregnancy, and they start to clean closets and sort through drawers, trying to make their home ready for the arrival of the baby. It's probably not a good idea to do something as strenuous as scrubbing floors in your last week of pregnancy, so try to confine the nesting instinct to lighter chores. You should be getting rest and saving your energy.

6. Effacement Beginning. Your cervix will start to thin. You won't feel the change, but your doctor or midwife will comment on this during your examination.

(You'll be making more frequent visits during your last month of pregnancy.)

*7. **Bloody Show.*** The mucus plug lodged in your cervix, which adds another barrier of protection for the fetus, may dislodge before you go into labor. You might find it in your underwear or see it in the toilet bowl. It simply looks like a blob of mucus tinged with a bit of dried blood. It is nothing to be alarmed about; it's simply a sign that your labor is nearing. If you're already contracting regularly, it means that you're probably in labor.

*8. **Ruptured Membranes.*** Everyone has heard of the woman who "breaks her water," and we have images of standing in the middle of a supermarket or sitting in someone's house at a dinner party and suddenly finding ourselves soaking wet and in labor. This will not necessarily happen. Your membranes may or may not rupture ahead of time; if they do not, your physician may rupture them artificially before delivery. This does *not* hurt. Or your water may break ahead of time, either before or during your early labor. If your water breaks, you may not have a gush of water but rather only a trickle, as the baby's head may be pressing down into the pelvis and blocking the flow.

Whether you have a trickle or a flow, call your doctor. Many doctors do not want you to wait more than twenty-four hours before labor begins after the rupture of membranes and may want to induce your labor. The baby is more susceptible to infection without the protection of the membrane and fluid. Also, you will be told not to bathe, but rather to take a shower.

You may not be sure, if you only have a trickle of fluid, whether your water has broken. One way you might know is that amniotic fluid, unlike urine, is colorless and odorless. It used to be thought that breaking your water ahead of time, what was once called a dry birth, would make childbirth more difficult, but this is not the case; your body replaces all of that fluid within three hours. You may find, however, that breaking your water in early labor may seem to advance the labor along. Your contractions may become stronger, closer together, and more regular.

9. False Labor. You've all heard stories about women coming to the hospital only to be told they're not really in labor, would they please go home and wait. Although getting sent home from the hospital is covered in the next chapter, a few words should be said here about false labor. It can be Braxton Hicks contractions, coming close together and masquerading as labor, or it could be early prodromal labor, which may involve contractions that become regular, get close together, and then, for whatever reason, stop.

They won't stop forever. Labor will eventually start—or start up again. Since you will be at home when your labor starts, you are not in a position to know if you're in labor except by the strength and regularity of your contractions. With first babies, this is particularly difficult to judge. Many, many women—including doctors' wives and even doctors—show up at the hospital who are experiencing what is called false labor, so don't feel embarrassed or concerned if you happen to take false labor seriously.

One way you can tell you're in labor is that real labor doesn't stop or go away, it just keeps getting more intense. As it becomes stronger, it interferes with sleep. If you find yourself napping in the middle of your "labor," you're probably not *in* labor. With real contractions that are coming steadily and getting progressively stronger, you won't be able to talk or laugh or joke during one.

Of the three stages of labor, the first is what people commonly associate with the actual word "labor," which literally refers to the work of childbearing. The first stage, called the stage of dilatation, begins with the first signs that you are ready to have your baby and ends with the moment when your cervix is fully dilated and you are ready to push the baby out during what is called expulsion. The second stage, the stage of expulsion, is when the baby is pressed down into the birth canal and then delivered. The third stage, the stage of the placenta, is when the placenta is expelled.

The first stage of labor is made up of four parts, and this is what will be discussed during the rest of this chapter. This is the stage that is most frequently feared, and about which, oddly enough, most women know the least.

The beginning of the first stage of labor is known as the *prodromal* part of labor. This is when labor is just beginning. During this part, labor is the easiest. For many women, this is the longest stage. It can, in fact, last up to several days. In some women, this part is skipped entirely. For those of you who have already had babies, this part probably will not exist. It is during this part of labor that the cervix does most of its thinning, or effacement. In order for the cervix to open up to admit the baby through, it must thin out from its long and closed state. This process can be very slow for some people. During this time, the contractions are very irregular and may be very brief. You're not even sure you're in labor. The pattern of contractions is very hard to predict. One may come in five minutes, the next in ten, the next in three, the next in twenty. While there may be effacement taking place, there is usually very little dilatation happening at this time. The contractions may not hurt at all, or they may be a bit painful. During this part of labor, your contractions may even stop for several hours, then resume. Toward the end of this part of labor, the contractions may become more regular and more predictable.

Your mood during prodromal labor will be very excited, as you begin to anticipate what will be happening to you. You may also begin to get a bit frightened and you probably will not be able to sleep, though if you can, please do. You'll need all the rest you can get for what lies ahead.

This is a good time to start your relaxation. Lie down or sit in a chair, whatever is comfortable, and relax. The more you relax, the better you will feel. You probably won't need your breathing right away. Conserve your energy, since this part of labor may last for quite a long time.

Prodromal labor is the time to do some of the things you'll want to get accomplished before you leave for the hospital. Finish packing your bag. Before the contractions get too strong, take a shower, shave your legs, put on deodorant. Don't put on a lot of makeup in anticipation of being the most glamorous patient in labor that the hospital has ever seen. Many women come in with mascara, makeup base, and blusher on. Within a half hour, the mascara has run down their faces in great black streaks and the makeup and blusher are itchy with perspiration. If you feel you can't go anywhere without some makeup on, stick to lip gloss, which will keep your lips moist when they have a tendency to dry, and a bit of vaseline on your eyelashes. Keep your hair simple, too. If it's long, tie it back with an elastic band or pin it back with barrettes. A plastic headband, the kind with teeth, is also a good idea to keep your hair off your face. Glamorous hairstyles end up in wet strings hanging over your face.

If you think you're in labor, even early labor, don't eat any heavy meals. In fact, when your contractions are regular, don't eat any solids at all. Stick to clear fluids. You can prepare some Jell-O ahead of time; it's okay to eat that during early labor. If you've been in prodromal labor a while and are feeling starved, call your doctor and check with him. Remember that even if you are hungry, eating may cause you a great deal of discomfort, and may even cause nausea and vomiting. A lot of people in early labor get sent home from the hospital and think that is the green light for food: they eat double cheeseburgers, french fries, malteds. When they return to the hospital, as they all do within a certain number of hours, they throw up on the nurses. So please, no food in labor—for our sake as well as yours!

If you happen to have a long prodromal labor, the worst side effect can be exhaustion. After a day or two, you'll feel very fatigued. This can put you at a disadvantage for the rest of the labor that is to come. Don't get too excited if things are going slowly; use the extra time to relax. Try to catch short naps.

The second part of the first stage of labor is known as the *latent* phase. During this part of labor, there isn't much question whether you're in labor or not. This part of labor usually lasts about two to six hours. The contractions are much better defined and are more regular. They may not last much longer than the contractions you had during prodromal labor, but they'll be stronger. Keep relaxing. You don't even have to start your breathing until you feel you need it. You should also stay at home unless you're too uncomfortable. (If you can still relax and you're not making faces and squinting, or holding your breath, or gripping the arms of your chair, you don't need your breathing yet. If you're doing any of the above, start your breathing. Start with the slow chest breathing.)

This is usually the part of labor during which your effacement is completed and you dilate one to four centimeters.

Memo to the Coach

Remember that being in labor, prodromal or latent, doesn't mean that the woman has to curl up on the bed just because she decides she wants to start the breathing. In fact, in the early stages of labor it might be even better for the woman to walk around. Remember too that before she begins any breathing exercises, or before she decides to switch from one form of breathing to the next in the progression, she should change her position first.

Your mood during this part of labor is still very excited, but since you recognize that this is really labor, you become more businesslike.

If you decide to use your breathing, remember to use the focal point and get into a comfortable position. Effleurage can also be helpful with the breathing in these early phases. Make your motions slow and gentle. Rest as much as you can between contractions. If you're really tired, this is still a good time to try to catnap between contractions. It is also the time when you want to have your coach by your side, or at least to inform him you're in labor and start him on his way home. As for calling your doctor, ask your physician or midwife ahead of time exactly when he or she wishes to be informed. You will receive specific instructions as to when to telephone.

Memo to the Coach

You may have trouble getting her to relax now. She's getting excited, but she mustn't forget the need for relaxation, so employ your stroking between and during the contractions. Time the contractions if they seem to be getting closer together.

You should be able to do your breathing on your own during this phase, so if your coach is tired or it's the middle of the night, it's a good idea to let him get as much rest as possible. You'll need the coach awake and energetic later on.

In these early parts of labor, don't get too hung up on timing the contractions. All you need is a general idea of how close together they are. A military officer whose wife was in prodromal labor for three days kept a three-ringed notebook by his side and painstakingly recorded every single contraction for seventy-two hours. When he arrived at the hospital, he proudly handed his log over to the nurses, who tossed it aside. He was crushed. Don't waste your time. When the contractions seem to be less than five minutes apart, you can concern yourself with timing them. But it isn't necessary to write anything down.

CHAPTER TEN

Time to Get Serious: Active Labor and Transition

The *active* part of labor is next, and by this time, most people are in the hospital or on their way there. From contracting every five to ten minutes, you'll be having pains every three to five minutes, and they'll be very well defined. This part of labor lasts two to six hours, and it basically encompasses the dilatation of the cervix from approximately five to seven centimeters. Once the cervix has been fully effaced, as it should be during the latent part of labor, you will generally dilate at the rate of approximately one centimeter per hour. The last centimeters usually go faster than the first ones. Your contractions will last about one minute each and will be more sharply defined and intense. The peaks of the contractions will be much longer, and you'll have to work harder than you did during the latent phase.

Your mood will be very serious, you'll be working harder, and you may find your confidence wavering a bit as the contractions get stronger. Progress with your breathing as you need it, remembering to change your position before you switch breathing techniques. Modified chest breathing with shallow breathing at the peaks is good during active labor, as is accelerated-decelerated shallow chest breathing. Beware of hyperventilation with the shallow breathing. Remember your cleansing breaths, always, and use your focal point.

Be aware of the possibility of *back labor*. It can become very uncomfortable for some women, especially during this part of labor and on to delivery. Most women have their babies in an anterior position during labor—that is, with the baby's head toward the front of the body. The baby is born looking at the floor in this position. But some women have their babies in a posterior position (*Figure 27*) during labor and even during delivery, with the back of the baby's head pointing toward the woman's back and the head pressing into her lower back during each contraction. The baby is born, then, looking up at the ceiling. This kind of labor can be slower and more painful, because you may feel the contractions only in your back.

During labor, some babies will rotate to an anterior position (*Figure 28*) on their own, but if they don't and if you are having back labor, the most helpful thing to do is to have the coach apply direct massage to your back.

Changing position will also help. Get off your back. Lie on your side or get up on all fours (*see Figure 29*). That makes the weight of the baby fall forward, and it

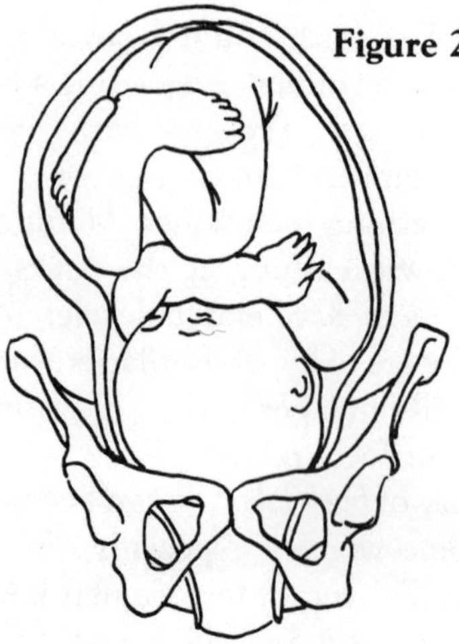

Figure 27: Posterior Position

Figure 28: Anterior Position

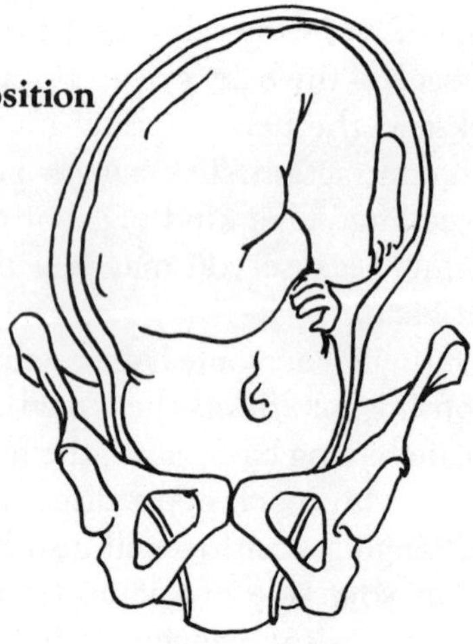

helps tremendously with the pain. It can also help the baby to rotate to the preferred position. You might also try leaning forward onto the back of a chair (*see Figure 30*).

Memo to the Coach

Put the heel or palm of your hand (the heel might be better) directly on the spot that is most painful and exert counterpressure. Don't be afraid: press as hard as you can! As you massage, rotate your hand in a circular motion. Some people use a tennis ball, pressing it in and rubbing it on the painful spot.

Since you're working very hard and concentrating very hard, using effleurage during this part of labor may be distracting. As soon as you find yourself losing concentration while you're doing it, immediately stop the massaging. It's important to be flexible about what you're doing. And speaking of being flexible, be especially aware now that you should be using whatever breathing helps you get through. Don't skip way ahead to an advanced kind if you haven't tried the ones in between; you don't want to leave yourself at the end with no further breathing techniques to use. But *don't* say, "Well, I'm in active labor now, so I guess I ought to move from the slow chest breathing to something more complicated." Whatever works for you is what's good. And 99 percent of the time at any given moment of your labor you won't even know what phase you're in. You aren't examined very

Figure 29:

Getting down on all fours is one of the best positions for relieving low backache and for reducing pressure on the spine.

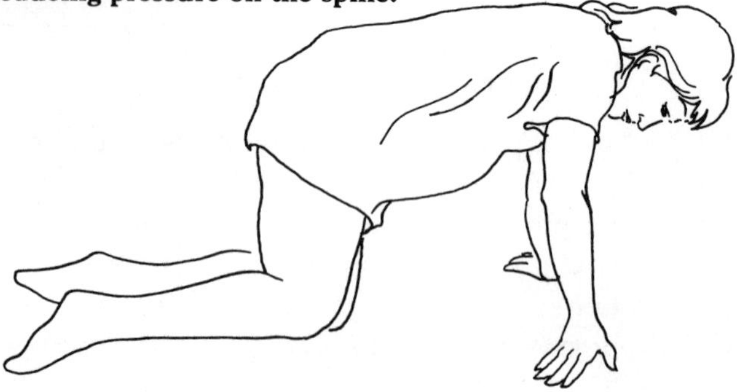

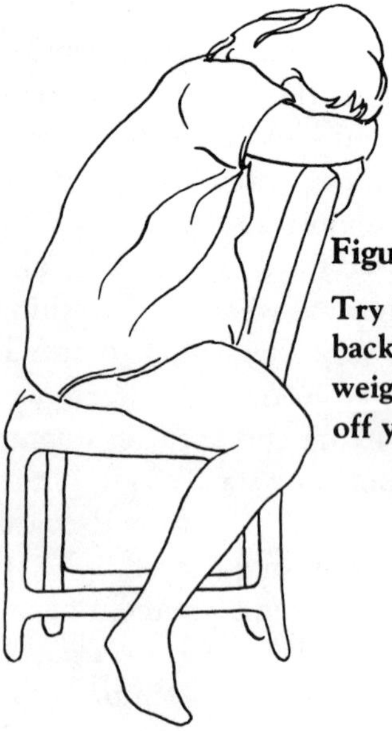

Figure 30:

Try leaning forward onto the back of a chair, so that the weight of the baby is lifted off your spine.

often, and you can only guess how dilated you are. So quit worrying about where you are and apply your breathing as you need it.

Memo to the Coach

In active labor, look for signs that the breathing she's using isn't working. Watch for grimacing, clutching, squeezing of hands, of blankets, or bed rails. Get her to try to increase the rate of the breathing she's doing and to change her position if you think it's not working. If she hasn't been examined in a long while, ask for a doctor or midwife to take a look. She may be a lot further along than either of you thinks. Or she may be progressing very slowly and becoming exhausted. This is the time when you may want to make a decision about anesthesia. (Various types of anesthesia and pain medication will be discussed extensively in Chapter 14.) If she wants anesthesia, be supportive of her decision. Help her evaluate her situation but remember that you don't want to make her feel discouraged. Think positively. You'll be helping her during this time with various comfort supports—cool washcloths, ice chips, sour lollipops. Reinforce relaxation; it's much harder to get her to relax now, but you have to try. And change into your scrub suit before she's fully dilated.

Transition, the last part of the first stage of labor, can be the shortest of all the phases. It signals that the end is near. It can also be the hardest to get through due to its intensity. It lasts from one to three hours (or sometimes longer), and during this time your cervix will go from seven centimeters to a fully dilated ten centimeters. The contractions become more erratic and harder to predict in terms of intensity and duration. Some may have double peaks; just when you think the contraction has peaked and is subsiding, it may begin to peak again. They can last from sixty to ninety seconds and be two to three minutes apart. The breathing is extremely difficult here, partly because of the intensity of the contractions and partly because it's much more difficult to concentrate. More people will come bustling in and out of the labor room as you get toward the end.

You may have as little as half a minute between the contractions to rest. Still, you must try to relax and rest during each interval. This is a good place to use the puff/blow breathing. If you're having difficulty concentrating, your coach can signal you to switch from 3/1 to 2/1 to 1/1. Watching his signals can force you to concentrate harder. It makes you think about what you're doing, and during transition that's helpful. You will also feel a strong urge to push toward the end of transition; *do not push* until you get the okay to do so from your doctor. The baby's head is down very low at this time, exerting a great deal of pressure. Using the puff-and-blow breathing, especially one puff and one blow during the times when you feel like pushing most, will help you curb that urge.

Your mood during transition may run the gamut of some rather unpleasant emotions. You may be agitated, overwhelmed, discouraged. You may even panic, become paranoid, lose your perception. You may be irritable and even extremely angry.

Memo to the Coach

Do not leave her now. If you have to change into a scrub suit for the delivery room, do it before transition. Don't go to the bathroom now, or step out for a cup of coffee. She needs you most at this time. Your encouragement is more important here than at any other time. Tell her she's doing great, that she shouldn't give up, that she should hang on in. If she's having trouble with the breathing, do it with her. This may be a good time for her to use your face as a focal point. Get her to stare at you and do the puffs and blows together. This can be immensely helpful. Don't let her lose control. And try to get her to rest between contractions.

Women have been known to curse wildly, beg for divorces, swear off sex forever, and throw things at their husbands during transition. Physically, you may be feeling less than in control due to episodes of nausea, vomiting, sweating, chills, and trembling. Only some or maybe even none of these things may apply to you, but it's a good idea to recognize just how difficult this part of labor can be. It's better not to underestimate the downside. It's not dangerous, but it is exhausting. Encouragement and eye-to-eye contact can save the day here. Labor nurses sometimes climb right up onto the bed and breathe along with women who claim they just can't make it any further. And it works!

After transition you will be ready to push and then to

have your baby delivered. Somehow, by keeping in mind the fact that you are near the end, you will be able to get through the hardest part.

The first stage of labor, as described here, is based on an average labor: what will happen to most of the women who have children but not all. It must be emphasized that your labor may differ from the labor we have outlined in one or in many ways, from the duration of each part of labor to the length and intensity of your contractions, to the discomfort experienced during transition, to your feelings and emotions. But two things are sure—you *will* pass through these phases in the order in which they are listed, and, after the next stage of labor, you *will* have your baby.

While you're waiting at home, remember the following fundamentals:

1. Drink only fluids. Don't eat anything solid.
2. Be relaxed.
3. Conserve your energy.
4. Don't prescribe your own medicine. Don't try to give yourself an enema or take a laxative (unless your doctor tells you to do so).
5. Don't get hung up on timing your contractions.

Try to look ahead to what is going to happen to you with an open mind. Don't let any fears take over. You'll be prepared; you'll know what to expect. The next hours may be the most exciting and significant in your life, and you'll want to remember them always as a time of positive feelings.

CHAPTER ELEVEN

General Hospital: Advance Preparation

There is no hard and fast answer to the question, When should I go to the hospital? Frankly, you'll go when you want to go, regardless of what anyone tells you. But here's some good advice: don't go to the hospital too quickly. As long as you're not in agonizing pain, as long as you're not desperately uncomfortable, stay home. Unless you live an hour from the hospital or there's a blizzard or a transit strike, stay put. Once you get to the hospital, you'll have to cope with whatever procedures you've decided on or your doctor requires—such as enemas, I.V.'s, blood tests, monitors. Hooked up to a monitor and an I.V., you'll have to stay on your bed, and in early labor, walking might be more comfortable for you.

If you have any questions about when to go to the hospital, be sure to ask your doctor ahead of time. Babies are notorious late-night visitors, and many a labor begins in the wee hours of the morning. You may not want to disturb your doctor or midwife when the time comes, so ask in advance.

It's also nice to make a list of all the things you'll need, both for the labor room and for your hospital room after delivery. Here's what we suggest you pack:

During Labor

The prepared childbirth bag should be a separate tote containing the following aids:

Sour lollipops (three or four). Your mouth will get very dry, and you may have a bad taste there. The lollies are good for energy because of their sugar, and they will aid your saliva flow because of their tartness.

Tennis balls. They will help with the pain of back labor. Press them into the most painful spot and massage with circular motion.

Talcum powder. Your skin may get chafed during effleurage or back massage. Powder will soothe these areas, and it will help refresh you when you're feeling sweaty.

Lip balm. Your lips will get dry from your breathing, especially shallow chest breathing; you won't be permitted to drink, except for sucking on ice chips provided by the hospital. Lip balm soothes chapped lips.

Mouth spray. A small purse-sized container will rid your mouth of a bad taste.

Sweat socks. Many women find that their feet get very cold during labor because they're sweaty and chilled. Hospitals don't supply socks, so bring your own.

Pillow. The hospital gives you one pillow; you may want a second to prop up your knees or feet, or to put under your behind. Don't bring your best pillowcase; it can get messy during childbirth.

Picture or object for focal point. Make sure it's portable; even though you're attached to it, if it's cumbersome it won't do.

Washcloth. Your own washcloth, which will be soothing when dampened with cool water, will be considerably softer and fluffier than the hospital's.

Bands or barrettes for hair. You'll want to tie or pin your hair back if it's long or if it hangs down on your face.

Snack for coach. Pack a sandwich, fruit, cookies, a small can or bottle of juice, and perhaps a candy bar or other energy food.

Crib notes. If you're afraid you won't remember all the breathing sequences, write down some notes on a small pad or some index cards so you or your coach can consult them.

Telephone numbers and dimes. Get a roll of dimes from the bank and make a list of everyone you'll want to inform about the good news.

Camera. If you're willing and he's inclined, the coach can take pictures of you in labor or giving birth. Be sure, though, that he doesn't get so busy with the camera that he forgets his role as coach.

Champagne. Why not?

Hot-water bottle or dry ice pack. The water bottle may help soothe during back labor. Dry ice packs are available in some stores; they are self-contained and when opened, become cold and can be applied to painful areas.

Memo to the Coach

It should be your responsibility to remind her not to pack any money or valuables in her bags, or to take any with her when you go to the hospital. There is no way to safeguard your property at any given moment, so it's best to leave these things behind. Anything she wants with her can be brought to the hospital after the birth of the baby.

After Labor

You should have a separate suitcase for the personal things you'll need during your hospital stay. These should include:

Robe. Bring a pretty, long, washable robe that you can wear for visitors or for classes on how to bathe the baby. You'll be bleeding quite a bit after childbirth, so don't bring anything too fancy or not washable, like silk.

Slippers. Pack a pair without much of a heel, since you may not be very comfortable walking right away. Backless styles are a good idea.

Socks. If your feet get cold at night.

Nightgowns. Not your best. You may want to stay in your hospital gowns and cover them with your robe. If you want your own nightgowns, bring some inexpensive, washable styles or some older ones you're not too attached to. Remember, if you're going to nurse, they should unbutton in front.

Underpants. You'll be wearing a sanitary pad and belt provided by the hospital. You'll want to put underwear over this. It's a good idea to use your own maternity underwear, since you won't be needing it afterward.

Going-home outfit. Bring a maternity outfit or a loose-fitting, chemise-style dress; you won't fit into your old clothes right away. Bring accessories you'll need for this outfit.

Bras. Bring maternity bras or bras that open in front if you're going to nurse, tight-fitting bras with good support if you're not.

Cosmetics. Small sizes of the products you like are best; they're sold in many drugstores. Also pack toothbrush, toothpaste, brush and comb, your own soap if you're very fond of it, hair dryer, and a razor.

Makeup. You'll want to look terrific for all your visitors, and for yourself, so pack the works—blusher, makeup base, eyeliner, lipstick, perfume, hair accessories, astringent, moisturizer, cotton swabs, cotton balls, nail polish, polish remover, emery boards.

Outfit for the baby to go home in. A receiving blanket, stretchy, sweater, hat, whatever is appropriate for the season.

Books. This is a perfect time to read those books on nursing your baby or child care that you've bought; magazines and newspapers can be nice, too.

Pad and pen. Good for writing down phone numbers for callbacks (you may be nursing when a friend or relative calls), as well as to note who sent telegrams, flowers, candy, balloons. If you're very organized, you can bring thank-you notes to write for in-hospital gifts.

Radio, bedside clock, tape cassettes and recorder. Try to make yourself as comfortable as possible. Remember: you'll be in the hospital, but you won't be *sick.*

Polaroid camera. If you have one, or can borrow one, it's a great idea for instant snaps of the new baby and parents.

There are many discussions that you should have with your doctor or midwife well before you check in. First, make sure that your doctor agrees with you if you want a natural childbirth or that you see eye to eye about anesthesia. If your physician practices in a partnership or a group, make sure the other doctors agree with you as well. You don't want to argue with someone when you're in active labor. Tell them your choices, let them express their opinions, and meet on common ground ahead of time.

If the group practice is a large one—more than three doctors, for instance—make certain you have met all the doctors and spoken with them at least once before the due date. Remember, it's your body and your baby. But also keep in mind that there are good reasons for doctors and midwives to feel the way they do on certain subjects, so be prepared to listen to them.

After you and your doctor see eye to eye on the big issues, you'll also want to bring up some smaller ones—whether or not to have an enema, the use of an intravenous line, what kind of prepping (shaving) the doctor wishes to do, what kind of anesthesia he favors if you need it, what kind of pain-relieving drugs he might use, the kind of incision he'll do for a Cesarean, how late he'll let you go past your due date before inducing labor, and whether he prefers the birthing room (if the hospital has one) or the labor room. All of these issues will be discussed here in full, so you can ask informed questions. But do remember that you are entitled to have your preferences about these procedures.

There are, as well, certain obstetrical procedures you can discuss ahead of time, but these are the physician's choice; in other words, you can't object to what he's doing since it may be for the well-being of the baby. But you can ask ahead of time and find out what he favors. These areas include whether he uses forceps frequently, what he feels about whether or not you should have an episiotomy, when he feels a Cesarean is necessary. You can discuss these areas with him in advance, but you cannot insist on having your way. These are medical decisions.

It's a good idea as part of your advance preparation to take advantage of the hospital tour, which most institutions have and which some prepared childbirth groups sponsor. Schedule your tour well before your due date. You'll find it will make a big difference in your approach to childbirth; you'll have seen your physical surroundings, and you'll feel less afraid of the unknown. Procedures will be explained to you then, so you won't have to worry about what the hospital will expect when you arrive in labor.

Now you're ready to go to the hospital. You're in pretty active labor; your contractions are regular and have begun to make you feel quite uncomfortable. Before you leave home, call your doctor and let him know you're going to the hospital. He will then phone the hospital and tell them. Now you pick up your suitcase and your prepared childbirth bag and you walk out the door.

CHAPTER TWELVE

That's Why They Call It Labor: The Labor Room

The first obstacle you'll encounter when you get to the hospital is admissions. Many women fear that they will be trapped in admissions for hours and required to fill out a multitude of forms, but there's no reason to worry about this. Almost all hospitals have preadmissions for obstetrical patients precisely so you won't get stuck in the waiting room. If admissions *does* seem to be taking a long time, just turn around and head for the labor floor yourself. They'll always be able to track you down later and find out your mother's maiden name. (There's only been one case that we know of where the admissions office turned into a delivery room, and that occurred when a woman had been sent home because she wasn't in active labor. She waited a bit too long before she returned to the hospital.) There's no reason to fear a snafu; checking in at admissions should take only a few minutes.

After you've been admitted, you'll be taken up to the labor suite. This is one of the few times when a woman and her coach might be separated. The coach will be sent to put on a gown while you're settled in your room. This is done so that strange men don't walk into shared labor rooms and stumble upon another woman in labor. The woman in the next bed has to be allowed some time to close her curtains and arrange herself. Also, some doctors don't like to examine the new patient with her coach standing next to them. But if you feel that your coach has been gone too long, speak up and request that he be allowed in. Labor nurses know that coaches are important; they won't try to keep you apart. In some hospitals, you will not be shown to your labor room or birthing room right away; these hospitals have separate examining rooms for new patients, where you're examined and assessed before being taken to your bed. Whether you will be admitted is determined then.

Getting sent home is seen as something of a trauma, but it needn't be; many women get sent home, and there's nothing wrong with spending a lot of your labor at home. You have freedom, mobility, and more distractions than you would have in a hospital. Prodromal labor can be very regular and quite painful and can seem like very active labor. But if it isn't and you're given the option to go home, *go home.* If you live very far from the hospital, go to a movie or go have a cup of tea. Eventually you'll notice a definite strengthening of the contractions.

Once you're in good, active labor and are progressing, you're admitted to the labor floor and the hospital routine begins. Sometimes you'll be alone at the beginning, but often your coach will be allowed in. You'll take all your clothes off except your socks (if you want to keep them on), and you'll put on a hospital gown. The labor nurse will check your blood pressure, your pulse, and your respiration and take your temperature. Once your vital signs are recorded, you'll be placed on a fetal monitor, which will keep track of the baby's heartbeat and of your contractions. You can be connected to the monitor in any of several ways. Some machines have a thin elastic band that you pull up over your legs onto your belly. Others have wide belts that go around the belly and fasten with Velcro. These are *external monitors.* They have two pieces that fasten onto you, superficially, on your skin. One is shaped like a cloverleaf and is placed on your lower abdomen. This picks up the baby's heartbeat and amplifies it so that anyone in the room can hear it. The other is a plastic piece placed higher on your belly with a button that gets pushed in as your uterus tightens. The machine then records the contractions on a paper printout.

It's important to know that this procedure is subject to your movement and to the baby's movement. If you turn on your side or change your position in any way, the monitor will stop picking up the baby's heartbeat. If the baby moves, it will also not pick up the heartbeat or contractions. The machine will stop making sounds or flitter uncontrollably, or a light will go on or a beep will sound. Don't be alarmed! This does not mean there is any problem.

Except in cases where it is essential to keep a close watch on the baby, due to the possibility of problems (see Chapter 15), it won't matter if the machine is temporarily interrupted. The presence of a monitor can be very inhibiting to many women in labor; they become afraid to move around (which is a natural desire in labor), because they don't want to interrupt the machine. But unless there is a problem, your being comfortable is more important than the monitor, so move all you want and ignore the short interruptions of the machine.

If it is necessary to watch the heartbeat of your baby and you want to be more comfortable, there is another way to record this information, and that is with an *internal monitor*. This is attached via a vaginal exam, in which a small electrode is placed onto the skin of the baby's scalp, very superficially, and a spiral wire then comes out of you and leads to a plate taped to your leg, which in turn has a wire leading to the monitor. You will then have freedom of movement while the recording of the baby's heart is taking place accurately.

Memo to the Coach

The monitor can be a great help to you, for you'll be able to see exactly when each contraction is beginning, peaking, and starting to go away. But don't get so hung up on the machine that you ignore your wife. One husband sat in front of the monitor as if it were a television set, and each time a contraction began, he would shout: "Here it comes! Another one's about to start! There it goes!" His wife, staring at her focal point and doing her breathing alone, replied through gritted teeth, "I know, shmuck!"

The monitor records your contractions, as well as the heartbeat. It indicates their duration—where each one begins and ends—and their frequency—where one begins and then where the next one begins.

After you're hooked up to the monitor, you'll be examined. It may not be right away, but fairly soon someone is going to give you a vaginal exam to determine if you're truly in labor and, if you are, how effaced and dilated you are. They'll also want to check the baby's position.

You'll be examined by a doctor, a nurse, a midwife, or, if it's a teaching hospital, a resident. Sometimes they like to examine you during a contraction to see what happens to the cervix and the baby's head while you're contracting. They use their hand: with their fingers, they can determine how dilated and effaced you are. Here they will employ a set of numbers to tell how far you have progressed. You can learn what the numbers mean and then, when you're examined, you can ask what yours are. You'll be told three things: how dilated you are (this is in centimeters), how effaced you are (this is a percentage), and what the station is, which refers to how far the head has descended into the pelvis. (This measurement is given in negative or positive numbers, from minus 4 to plus 4. The minus numbers are high in the pelvis; the plus numbers are low.) Thus, a person ready to deliver her baby would be 10 centimeters dilated, 100 percent effaced, and + 4 station.

During the exam, the doctor will perform what is known as Leopold's maneuvers, in which he or she will feel your abdomen in four specific places to find the baby's head, bottom, and sides. This examination can indicate if the baby is going to be either very large or very small. An approximate fetal weight is then determined.

The doctor is looking for signs of an extremely large baby or a date/size discrepancy. If you've been counting your pregnancy from the date of the last period you remember, and you've remembered wrong, you may be carrying a thirty-week baby and be in premature labor. This simple exam can help avoid surprises.

The doctor or midwife will also be checking to see if you've ruptured your membranes yet. If you have broken your water a day or two before, you may not be examined at all, due to the possibility of infection.

After your exam, if it's determined you're still in early labor, comes the enema, and this is when a lot of women get nervous. Some hospitals use a small Fleet enema; others use an enema bag. Of all the parts of labor and delivery, it's the one women express the most distaste for, perhaps because unlike their mothers and grandmothers, they have never had to experience an enema in their lives and they don't know what it's like. Also, if they have hemorrhoids, which many women do in late pregnancy, they're afraid it will hurt. Nurses in hospitals have a reputation for being great enema-givers; it's on all the greeting cards, a wizened old nurse with warts and missing teeth holding an enema bag and a bedpan, beckoning with one crooked finger.

This is how an enema is given; it's quite simple and fast. The nurse fills a bag with soapy water and tells the patient to lie on her left side, with her bottom knee straight and her right knee bent. The end of the rubber tube attached to the bag is lubricated; this is placed one and a half to two inches inside the rectum. The water is then let in, taking about a minute to empty completely. Then the tube is pulled out and the patient is asked to hold the water inside her until she has the urge to go to the bathroom.

Enemas do not stimulate labor, though it was once thought that they did. There's no real proof that they cause the contractions to intensify. An enema doesn't contaminate the delivery, either. And it is not the worst part of labor, despite what everyone fears. It is particularly good to have because if you do not have an enema, when it comes time to push, you may feel the urge to defecate and then you'll hold back on your pushing out of embarrassment. And you may well be embarrassed if you have an accident, which does often happen when no enema is administered. So, we recommend that you have an enema.

You will probably be hooked up to an intravenous line, because you cannot drink anything in labor, even water, and if you need anesthesia, any liquids could cause aspiration pneumonia, just as food might if vomited back up into the lungs. You can get very dehydrated during labor from sweating and breathing, and it's necessary to replenish those fluids somehow. An I.V. also contains sugar, which gives you and the baby energy, as well as electrolytes such as potassium and sodium that are lost during dehydration. You will need an I.V. for most anesthesia, and although it restricts your movement somewhat, you can still move around quite a bit if it's taped down well. Under most circumstances, though, you will not have an I.V. until you are in active labor. A needle to which a tube is attached is put into a vein and liquids can then drip through. It does not hurt.

You will also be shaved. Most hospitals no longer do a full prep (everything) but rather restrict the shaving to the perineum and part of the labia. This is known as the mini or partial prep. The reasons for the prep are that the hair could get caught in the stitches and can also make it harder for the doctor to sew you back up. It's easy and very quick and probably won't bother you very much; it's done with an ordinary plastic safety razor.

There will be blood drawn for a CBC (complete blood count), which will determine your red and white blood cell counts, your hemoglobin and hematocrit, as well as your Rh factor and blood type. These tests can determine if you have anemia or an infection, and they can indicate if you're bleeding. If you have a low blood count, the hospital blood bank must make sure they have your type of blood on hand, since a lot of blood is lost during delivery. Since your blood supply is virtually doubled during pregnancy and your uterus and its blood vessels are enlarged and engorged, you can bleed very fast. Even in the middle of the night, this blood is made ready.

If you haven't broken your water yet, this is probably the time when your membranes will be ruptured artificially. This is done only if your doctor or midwife is present. Membranes can be ruptured to attach an internal monitor to the baby's head or to determine if the fluid is clear. The breaking is done with a crochet hooklike tool and is completely painless. The doctor grasps the membrane between his fingers and snags it with the tool. All you will feel is warm fluid running between your legs.

At this time you will also be asked to sign consents for delivery and related procedures, which include Cesarean section, forceps delivery, and anesthesia. In the event of an emergency, no valuable minutes will be wasted with consent forms.

Once these procedures are completed, you will be left in your labor or birthing room with your coach. You'll have a labor nurse assigned to you, but she won't always be with you if everything's proceeding normally.

As your labor progresses and you're in more pain, it is extremely important to remember that you should never make *any* decisions during a contraction. If someone offered to sell you the World Trade Center during a contraction, you'd make a deal on the spot. You'd do anything. Always wait until the contraction ends, until the interval between the contractions, to talk. If anyone does try to talk to you during a contraction, ignore him or her.

Memo to the Coach

It's extremely important for you to realize that she is the one going through this, and that as much as you might want her to experience the birth without medication, you must be prepared to go along with what she wants. As long as she's not screaming to you in the middle of a contraction (during which she is not doing her breathing), you should take what she says seriously. Don't be like the guy reading the paper who said, as he read the sports pages, "Breathe, honey. You're not getting any painkillers." Then he lifted his eyes from his newspaper to tell the nurse, "I don't want my baby born sleepy." She might feel very guilty about needing anything, and your approval will be important. Be supportive.

And before you make any decisions, such as whether you want any pain medications or anesthesia, be sure to switch your position and try another breathing technique. Never simply decide you've had enough and quit on the spot. Try just a few times more, alternating what you're doing. It may be just what you need. If you haven't had a vaginal exam recently, you should also ask for one, because you may be much further along than you expected and might then decide not to have the anesthesia. Or you may be far slower, and the information will make your decision to ask for anesthesia that much easier.

As we approach the discussion of delivery, which will follow in the next chapter, it's a good time to bring up the subject of vanity, which is inevitably raised in all of our childbirth classes. No matter how prim and proper (and vain) you are, when it comes time for that baby to arrive, it's all going to hang out. You'll be more concerned about vanity before labor occurs than you will be during labor. Remember, you're going to be with professionals who have seen everything and are quite used to it.

Memo to the Coach

She'll be exposed and vulnerable, and there will be times when she won't realize it or care, so if you think she's exposed unnecessarily, be responsible: cover her up! If she wants the curtains closed, close them and keep them closed. It's up to you.

There are times when vanity and other considerations of personal appearance are thrust aside; sometimes this is due to the let-it-all-hang-out nature of childbirth. Other times, however, it's the craziness of the hospital that provides some of the most memorable moments. A nurse was told to expect the arrival of a new intern on the floor, a young doctor fresh from medical school whose name was Barry. The nurse was with a patient in labor who needed an examination. In walked a young man in a green scrub suit. "Are you Barry?" the nurse asked. He nodded. The nurse raised the sheet and parted the woman's legs. "Here," said the nurse. "Examine this patient." He gaped, then said, "How?" The nurse stared at him, thinking, Don't they teach them *anything* in med school these days? She handed him a plastic glove. "Put this on," she said impatiently. He pulled it onto his right hand. "Now what?" he said. "Examine her," the nurse demanded. "How do I do that?" he asked, puzzled. The nurse lost her temper. "For god's sake, don't they teach you doctors anything anymore?" "Doctor?" he replied. "Aren't you Barry?" the nurse asked. "Yeah," he replied. "Barry, the intern?" she said. "No," he answered. "Barry, the porter." Wham! The woman's legs slammed shut.

Just remember that when your time comes, if the door does swing open and the porter is mopping the corridor, you won't mind. You'll have other things to think about.

CHAPTER THIRTEEN

Push Comes to Shove: The Delivery Room

One night in Beverly Hills, California, after a posh dinner party, the guests were asked to assemble in front of a screen for some home movies. When they asked what they would be viewing, they were surprised to find out it wasn't a trip to the Greek islands or the host's and hostess's fifth anniversary party, but a film of the birth of their daughter. "Right in the delivery room," the hostess boasted, "in full color."

The movies rolled and the guests watched the hostess doing her breathing, relaxing during the intervals between contractions, sucking on ice chips, and in one shot, being coached by her husband. "Hey," one of the guests said, "if your husband's there next to you, who's taking the movies?"

"My *ex*-husband," the woman replied with a grin.

Obviously, delivery rooms can be the scene of some very interesting activities—aside from the birth of a baby. Despite their surgical ambience, they are not really very forbidding places. They are, in fact, the scene of much joy and happiness, and although they may look ugly to you when you go to visit them on your hospital tour, by the time your baby arrives, you'll probably think your delivery room is the most beautiful place on earth.

In most cases, you will be taken to the delivery room just before your baby is born. The first stage of labor culminates in the phase known as *transition*, in which the pains last the longest, are the strongest, and have the shortest interval between them. You may have passed through many different moods during transition; you may have felt hot and cold, shaky and paranoid, angry and hopeless. But although transition seems to be the worst part of labor, it is also the shortest. Your cervix is stretching just that last bit of the way to the point where it virtually melts away. The baby's head is pressing down quite hard, and you feel it very strongly in your rectum. (In fact, a sign that you are in the second stage of labor is that strong, unrelenting rectal pressure.) There's also a bit of bloody show at this point, due to the expulsion of a second mucus plug lodged higher in your cervix than the first. But although you may feel that you want to bear down and push, *do not push* until you are examined and given permission by the doctor or midwife. Pushing down on a less than fully dilated cervix can cause the cervix to swell, and with the swelling you lose all that ground you've gained in labor as the cervix dilates.

The second stage of labor, the stage of *expulsion,* begins with pushing and ends in the delivery room with the birth of the baby (or in a birthing room if that is what you have chosen). The most important thing about the second stage of labor—and the most difficult—is pushing. How to push is something that many women don't get quite right, and as a result they have to spend more time at it than they might have if they pushed correctly.

The hardest thing about pushing is that you will feel close to your limit at this point and now, after all you've been through, you're being asked to give everything you've got. (Doctors can be like football coaches: they don't let up until the baby has arrived!) It's hard to bear down in the right place; it's hard to keep your legs elevated; it's hard to concentrate.

Before we explain everything you always wanted to know about pushing, you should understand once again that you must not push until you are given permission to do so. One way of curbing the urge to push until you're ready is with blowing and panting. You need to hold your breath in order to push. (Try gently pushing with your rectal muscles without holding your breath and you'll see that it's necessary not to breathe.) By consciously breathing—and not closing your glottis—you will not push. (Your glottis, a flap of skin over your trachea, closes when your esophagus is used.) Since your birth canal is unstretched, you have to work hard to help your vaginal muscles. This part of your labor can take from one to two hours.

When the time does come for you to push, you will do so only during your contractions, pushing with them to help your body do its work. And pushing will make you feel better; it helps to relieve that strong urge you may have been feeling to bear down. (This is the stage during which having an enema pays off. Bearing down can cause urination and defecation. You don't want to be inhibited from pushing freely.) While you're pushing during your contractions, the baby is corkscrewing down the birth canal, performing the involuntary movements known as the cardinal movements of birth. The baby is helping, too.

Figure 31: The Pushing Position

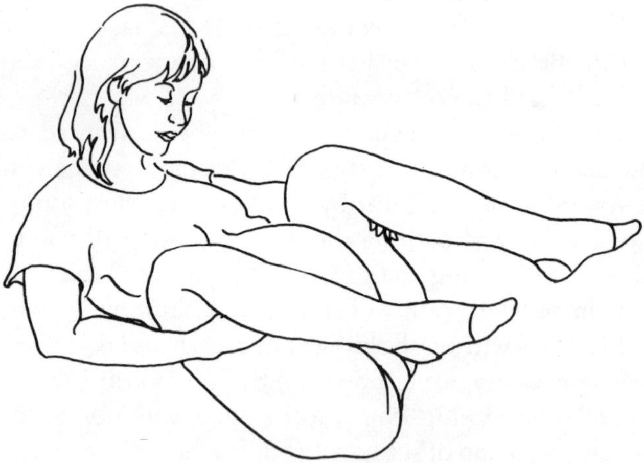

How to Push

Your head should be at a 35 to 40 degree angle; you won't be able to breathe properly if you're lying flat. You should not sit straight up either, because your pelvis curves, and this would force the baby to go uphill to be born. Your legs should be no more than 90 degrees from the flat of your body: remember not to compress your abdomen. (*See Figure 31.*) Keep your legs slightly apart and grab the inside of your thighs with your hands (you may also rest your legs on the bed rails or allow your legs to be held up by your coach or a nurse). It's important during pushing not to use your legs; to prevent that, your legs should be lifeless, propped up and out of the way. This also helps you to assume the natural position of your pelvis. Point your jaw down toward your chest to give you the maximum pressure on your rectum when you push. Push in your *rectum*, not in your legs, face, cheeks, shoulders, or chest.

Memo to the Coach

This is one of your big moments! Help make sure she's pushing correctly; if you see all the straining concentrated in her face, neck, and jaw, let her know. It's extremely important that the pushing be done properly. Help her to relax and concentrate her energy during the pauses between each push; she needs all the strength she can muster. And it is most important of all that you be present at this time; she needs you most. Don't go to the bathroom, step out for a cigarette, go to the pay phone. You should be there to offer her anything she needs—from encouragement, to ice chips to suck on, to a cool washcloth to sponge off her face.

This is a time when your Kegels will pay off: relax your perineum. Your legs and your jaw are relaxed as well.

You're ready to push. When you get a contraction, follow this breathing pattern:

Contraction begins. Take a cleansing breath. Then breathe in and push for 10 seconds. Let out the remaining air quickly. Take a long breath in, hold it and push again for 10 seconds. Let out the remaining air quickly. Take a breath in and push for 10 seconds. Let out the air and take a deep, cleansing breath.

You can practice this breathing and pushing ahead of time (but don't push hard, please—a gentle contraction of rectal muscles will do). Prop yourself up on a bed, or better still, lean back on your husband's knees when he's sitting and has his legs together and bent at the knee. Remember your cleansing breath at the beginning and at the end; remember, too, not to take much time between pushes. You don't want to lose time there because as you push, the baby is getting closer to delivery; and when you let up during a contraction, the baby slips back.

Another thing you want to remember about pushing is that you can be flexible. If the position described, propped up, lying back on the bed, is not comfortable for you during pushing and if you have the urge to squat or get on all fours, tell the nurse. Such positions can be accommodated, and women have been known to push more successfully when allowed their choice.

Pushing can take anywhere from a few minutes to two hours. Some factors that influence this—aside from how good you are at pushing correctly—are the size of the baby and its position. During this time your contractions will be coming every three minutes, which gives you a minute or two in between to relax. Make the most of that time. You have a lot of hard work ahead of you.

Finally, you will hear that the perineum is bulging,

which means that the very top of the baby's head, a bit of the hair perhaps, can be seen when you push. When the diameter of the head is visible during and after a contraction (called crowning), you will be moved from your labor room to the delivery room.

When the doctor says it's time to go to the delivery room, the nurse will take you off the fetal monitor and will bring your I.V. pole as she rolls your bed down the hall. Your coach will already have changed into his scrub suit (he's been told to do this before transition), and he will now be given a mask and cap and covers for his shoes. The doctor and nurse will mask and gown as well. You may be asked at some point during this transfer to stop pushing. Use panting to control the urge. You'll be moved from your bed to the delivery table, and your legs will be placed in stirrups. Your perineum will be placed on the edge of the bed, and as the doctor scrubs up, your perineum will be washed with an iodine solution. If you haven't been shaved yet, you may be shaved just a bit (the mini prep) now. The doctor will glove and gown.

Memo to the Coach

When the doctor takes over in the delivery room, you may feel you're just standing around. But you can still give encouragement and support. One warning—don't touch anything, or ask before you do so. No one wants sterile parts contaminated. If you feel faint, sit down. You don't have to stand and watch everything if you don't want to, but you can still take a place by her head and be there for support and to share the experience together.

You'll still be doing your pushing and breathing during these few minutes, unless you've been told not to push.

You'll be given a local anesthetic in your perineum or a pudendal block (which will be explained fully in the next chapter, on anesthesia), and the doctor will then ask you to push again, during which time your vaginal opening will be massaged to stretch it further. When there is enough tension on the perineum as the head bulges it outward, the doctor may perform an episiotomy—make an incision that prevents tearing. It will be done medially (lengthwise) or medialaterally (diagonally). A neat cut from the doctor, plus suturing, heals very nicely and is a great deal better than a tear.

Once the baby's head is born, the doctor will check to see if there's a cord around the baby's neck; you may be asked not to push while the cord is clamped or unraveled over the baby's head. The baby's nose and mouth will be cleaned out with a suction bulb and the head will turn to the side in a maneuver known as external rotation, so the baby's shoulders can pass through your birth canal one at a time, sideways. Once the shoulders deliver, the baby comes out quickly, and the doctor will clamp the cord and give you the baby (at last!).

Despite what you see on television, babies sometimes do not cry the instant the head comes out, so don't panic if yours doesn't. What's more, some babies look very different from what you might expect. Newborns are blue and wet, and their heads can be strangely shaped because of your pelvis (remember the Coneheads on *Saturday Night Live*?). If they're overdue, their skin may be peeling. If they're a bit premature, they may be covered with a whitish cream known as vernix, which protects them while they're floating in amniotic fluid. Their hands and feet may be very blue, and it may take quite a while before they pinken up. They may be bruised from forceps marks or from their birth experience. If a cord has wrapped around their necks, they may be blue in the neck and face. There might be some blood on their heads from the episiotomy (your blood, not theirs). Hair might be found growing on their shoulders and back, a remnant of the lanugo, or downy hair that covered them in the uterus. Their eyes may be swollen shut from birth. So when the doctor hands you this baby, don't be alarmed if any or all of these things are true. The Gerber Baby stage comes later.

Some doctors give the baby right to the mother, but many delivery rooms are very cool for the newborn. Since the baby is very wet when it appears, and since being cold can cause problems for babies, sometimes the newborns are given to the nurse and placed in the warmers kept in the delivery room until the nurse has dried them. If this occurs after your baby is born, remember that it's done for the baby's welfare. Newborns have inadequate temperature regulators and do not keep heat well. The nurse must also determine whether the baby needs suctioning, more stimulation for its respiration, or extra oxygen.

Some mothers like to try breast-feeding right away, in the delivery room, but we discourage that, since we've seen some unhappy results. First of all, lying flat on the delivery table makes it hard to breast-feed. Second, you're trying so hard to get your nipple in the baby's mouth that you might not even look at its face. Third, a less than perfect first time can get you uptight about further breast-feeding of your child, which is not a good way to begin. A better time to try breast-feeding, away from the glare and hustle of the delivery room, is in the recovery room, where you and your husband and the baby will be together for a bit more time right after the birth.

The nurse will wipe your baby off and wrap it in a blanket. Then, depending on where you're having your baby, she will give the baby a shot of penicillin or put silver nitrate in its eyes, precautions for venereal disease, and a shot of vitamin K to aid in blood clotting. Then the baby will be footprinted, and two hospital bands will be attached—one to its wrist, the other to its ankle. A third band, matching the baby's, will be attached to your wrist.

Nurses are required to give the baby two Apgar scores, one at one minute after birth and one at five minutes after, as a way of assessing the baby's well-being. There are five categories on which the baby is scored, with two points given in each category: color, respiration, heart rate, reflexes, and tone. Most babies do not receive perfect scores of 10 either at one minute or at five, because it is normal for a newborn to have blue hands and feet. In fact, the baby's hands and feet may not be as pink as the rest of it for a few days. One of the problems mothers create for themselves is that they come to regard the Apgar scores as a kind of early I.Q. test and spend their postpartum time comparing scores with other mothers. Anything above a 7 at 5 minutes means you've got a good baby. The Apgar score is, however, basically a tool for doctors and nurses, and in many cases no one volunteers the numbers to you.

One of the most important parts of our job is to determine the Apgar score. A timer goes off in the operating room at one and five minutes to remind us that we should be making these observations. They should not be subjective, nor should they have to bring in memories which may be hazy in recall later (now, let's see, how did the baby look at one minute?).

One thing about working in the delivery room that's difficult to describe is the pace. From the moment a woman is brought in, ready to deliver, until she is taken to the recovery room, the nurses and doctors move very quickly. The things we are describing—scrubbing up, episiotomies, delivery, cleaning the baby—all take place in very few minutes. People move double-time, and there's almost no chance to stop and think about what is happening.

The pace doesn't lessen after the baby arrives, because in addition to cleaning the baby and seeing to its well-being, there's another stage of labor yet ahead for the mother. This is the delivery of the placenta, or afterbirth, as it is sometimes known. After nine months of growth, of nourishing the fetus, the placenta is ready for its own delivery. You'll feel another contraction within five to twenty minutes, and the doctor will deliver this miraculous organ. If you have the chance, ask the doctor if you can take a look at your placenta. On the side that's been attached to the baby, you can see all of the blood vessels that brought fluids, oxygen, and nourishment to the growing fetus.

Most hospitals dispose of the placentas in various ways—for various brands of shampoo, for instance. There have been a few cases of people wanting to keep the placenta. The one we remember best was a husband who was rather vocal in his desire. His wife had had a Cesarean section, and he had waited outside the delivery room. After the birth, he went to the head nurse and requested his wife's placenta. He was told that the placenta had been thrown out. He became angry and said that the placenta was part of his wife's body, and if you had a leg amputated, you had to sign a form regarding disposal of that leg, didn't you? The nurse phoned the hospital administrators, who said that under no circumstances were placentas to be taken home by anybody. "It's hospital property," the head nurse told the husband, who in turn said he'd sue. After almost an hour of this discussion the nurse had had enough, so she went into the delivery room, retrieved the placenta from another recent birth, shoved it into a plastic garbage bag, and gave it to the man. "It wasn't his wife's," she said later, "but I don't think he'll know the difference." No one was sure why he wanted the placenta so much.

What we have described in this chapter is a childbirth without any interference. You may want anesthesia; you may need a Cesarean; there may be some small problem or difficulty. These things will be covered in the following chapters. No one has a labor and delivery that goes "by the book," and you shouldn't expect yours to. Everyone's labor is different; there is really no way to categorize a "typical" labor, so you must be prepared for anything to happen. Take the information in the following chapters into account and learn everything you can about what might occur. Only by learning what lies ahead will you feel secure and in control, no matter what path your labor follows.

CHAPTER FOURTEEN

No Thank You, Dr. Lamaze: Anesthetics and Analgesics

A woman is wheeled into the delivery room. She's just had an epidural (a regional anesthesia that results in no pain felt below the waist). She is placed on the table, and as she stares up at the giant arc light beaming down overhead, she breaks into a big grin. "That lamp is terrific!" she says. "Tell me where I can get one for my apartment."

That is a happy anesthetized patient.

Another woman has just had her baby after having the same epidural, and as she tries to get her newborn son to look at her, she exclaims, "He won't look at me! He's mad at me because I had an epidural. He doesn't like me.

Are you mad at your mother because she had anesthesia?"

That is an unhappy anesthetized patient.

Some women regard anesthesia as the only way to have a baby. "Are you crazy? This is the 1980s. Why should I suffer when modern medicine can take over? Besides, I won't be able to stand the pain." And some are gung-ho for natural childbirth and think the dirtiest word in the English language is "anesthesia." (The second is "Cesarean.")

Nurses have to cope with all kinds of attitudes in the labor and delivery rooms, but none arouses more ire and charged feelings than anesthesia. People are misinformed about how it's administered and what it does, and often, during a difficult labor, they forget what they've been told by their doctor about what they can ask for. They just say, "Give me *something.*"

You should be informed in advance, and you should know what your choices are, but the fact is, it's impossible to decide in advance what you are going to do. How can you reject all anesthesia when you don't know what kind of labor you're going to have? Conversely, how can you walk into a labor suite at the very start of your labor and demand anesthesia, anticipating that you won't be able to make it?

The most important thing to remember about all forms of help, whether they are anesthetics (which remove pain) or analgesics (which help make the pain more bearable), is that they are available to you in the hospital. You may not want anything to help you through your labor, but if you should choose to have some assistance, you ought to know what you can ask for and what you'll get. Never make your decision before you need to. Your labor may be very slow and you may have to be induced, which almost always requires anesthesia. Or you may progress so quickly you won't even be given an epidural; it will be too late for it to take effect. Don't go in with the attitude that anesthesia is a dirty word; you may need something, and your opinions will make it harder to cope later. You want to aim for childbirth without guilt. Don't feel bad about *any* decision you make.

Anesthesia is different today from what it used to be. The anesthesia that got a bad name was something that passed from the mother to the fetus. It created sleepy babies and freaked-out mothers who couldn't remember having had a baby. A popular anesthetic was a combination of Demerol and scopolamine, which created something popularly known as twilight sleep. You weren't exactly asleep during this, and scopolamine made women say and do strange things. Some women have dim memories of childbirth; others remember nothing at all. Ether also used to be administered, and mothers used to sleep a day or sometimes two after its use. They missed their deliveries entirely.

These drugs caused disorientation in women who were given them; the babies would come out very sleepy and limp, like dishrags. At the time the drugs were administered, anesthesia was considered safe and the attitude toward pain was that no woman should suffer needlessly. There really wasn't any form of childbirth education then in widely popular use that might have enabled women to go through labor and delivery without help. It was only some years later that the notion of no anesthesia for the *baby*'s sake was brought forth.

Other anesthesia was subsequently developed, including some that did not knock you out totally. Spinal anesthesia was often used, in which the anesthetic was injected into the cerebrospinal fluid by needle, causing numbness below the site of the injection. The popular "saddle block" of years past, a low spinal anesthesia, caused numb legs and often bad headaches following birth. This was due to the fact that the spinal fluid leaked out, causing a change in the fluid's pressure. But spinal anesthesia was not continuous anesthesia. It had to be given again when the first dose wore off.

Epidural anesthesia, which seems to us to be the best and most helpful form of anesthesia for labor and delivery, solves some of the problems associated with other anesthetics. For one thing, it is continuous. For another, it does not affect the baby at birth. It leaves the mother awake and aware. And it does not cause headaches or other unpleasant side effects.

Among the choices you have for pain relief are those drugs known as analgesics. Analgesics take the edge off the pain and, in some cases, can even kill the pain for a few hours. They do this by affecting your central nervous system, raising your pain threshold, and altering your perception of pain. They affect your entire body, circulating through your bloodstream and crossing the placenta, though only mildly if not given in large dosage. Your senses are affected as well, and you become drowsy and sleepy. This can be a pleasant sensation for some and an unpleasant feeling for others. Some women enjoy the drowsiness after many long hours of labor, while others object to feeling drugged.

The most widely used analgesic is Demerol. A narcotic, it can be administered by being injected intravenously (through an I.V.) or intramuscularly (a shot in your behind). If it's intravenous, you'll feel it working within a minute or two; if intramuscular, it takes ten to fifteen minutes to start affecting you and will not be as strong as the I.V. dose (more Demerol crosses the placenta if it's given intravenously). The average dose is 50 to 100 milligrams. You may feel dizzy as the drug takes hold; the room may seem to be spinning. You may feel nauseous and may vomit. We try to give the drug slowly to prevent this reaction. The nauseated feeling and the dizziness will pass in a minute or two, and some people will feel relaxed and sleepy. Others may feel strange and not very pleasant.

Demerol allows you to sleep between contractions. You'll wake up only at the peak, when the contraction is at its strongest. In good, active labor most people cannot sleep straight through, and as a result, when you wake suddenly you may be confused and disoriented and have trouble doing your breathing properly. The drug lasts from one and a half to two hours. Doctors usually give one or two doses at most.

The good points about Demerol are that it can make you feel nice and relaxed, even a bit drunk, and this can help the woman who is having a hard time relaxing in labor. She may be tensing not only during contractions but in the intervals, and thus getting exhausted. Demerol will make her relax. It's especially good for rejuvenation between contractions, and the sleep you can get is good if you've had a long prodromal labor. Someone who has been up for two days and is still only effacing will find Demerol a lifesaver; you can get some sleep and begin fresh. Demerol is also good for people starting to fall apart toward the end of their labor. And, finally, Demerol is easy to administer. You don't need a trained person and special equipment to give a patient relief.

You can use Demerol in your labor to buy time. If you think you want anesthesia but aren't yet ready to commit yourself to the finality of, say, an epidural, you can take some Demerol and see if just a bit of pain relief was what you needed. Refreshed, you may want to go on without any further help. Or you may find the relief is exactly what you want and you can have an epidural as soon as the Demerol wears off.

The bad points about Demerol include the fact that it crosses the placenta and can cause sleepy babies, possibly those with breathing problems. Babies born after Demerol is administered are sometimes more lethargic at birth than other babies. Also, as we have pointed out, Demerol can make the mother feel sleepy, disoriented, and not in control. If it is given when labor is not well established, labor can slow down and stop.

A variety of other drugs may be available to you, including morphine, Phenergan (which can be mixed with the Demerol; it helps prevent vomiting and in addition boosts the effectiveness of the Demerol), and possibly the tranquilizer Valium. Most doctors don't use Valium much anymore, as it remains active in the baby following birth. Narcan can be given to reverse the effect of any narcotic, including Demerol. It works very quickly.

Regional anesthesia is used in childbirth when anesthesia is called for except for certain emergency situations when general anesthesia is administered (see the following chapter on problems and complications).

Epidural anesthesia is a regional block given by an anesthesiologist or nurse-anesthetist. It is done in such a way that it won't hurt you or the baby. It does not have any major side effects. It is given through a puncture in your back, and it takes the pain away from your waist down. It will not affect your sensory perception; it will not make you groggy, sleepy, or disoriented. And you will not be paralyzed after the anesthesia wears off. (You cannot imagine how many women are afraid that this is going to cause something permanent to happen to their spines. Epidurals are injected into the epidural space in front of your spinal column, into air, not spinal fluid. Thus, the headaches that accompany spinal anesthesia don't occur.)

The procedure is very simple. If you request anesthesia, the anesthesiologist will come into your room and will ask you some questions. Do you have any allergies? Do you have any problems or complications with your pregnancy? Have you ever had any anesthesia before? Have you had any back injuries or problems, such as a slipped disk? (These can make it difficult to give the anesthesia.) When he is finished taking a brief history, the anesthesiologist will see that you have an I.V. hooked up, if you don't have one already. An I.V. is necessary during anesthesia to prevent any severe drops in blood pressure. An epidural can cause your veins to dilate and your blood pressure to lower (hypotension). An increase in your fluids helps to prevent this. Sometimes the doctor will wait a bit while you get an extra bottle of fluid inside you before he starts the procedure.

The anesthesiologist will then explain what he's about to do. You then have to agree to it, and may be asked to sign a written consent. Nothing will be done if you don't want it. Listen carefully and ask any questions you may have. When you have given your consent, the doctor will ask you to roll on your side and come to the edge of the bed. Your back will be facing him. You will then assume a fetal position by bringing up your knees and bending your head down. The bottom part of your spine, your lower back, will curve out naturally in a bow shape. Since the doctor will be working in the space between your bones, the more you curve, the bigger that space gets and the easier it is for him to find it. Some doctors will ask you to sit up and bend your head down, but the idea is the same: when your back curves, the bones separate.

He will then wash your back off with an iodine solution. You will feel a cold and wet sensation. This is necessary because it is a sterile procedure. He will then put a sterile towel on your back. It is important not to move while he does this, to stay as still as you can—which may be hard while you're having contractions.

When the doctor feels the right spot, he will give you an injection of a local anesthetic similar to Novocain (which feels like a bee sting followed by an instant of a burning sensation), and once the skin and surrounding ligaments are anesthetized, he will begin. He will put a needle into your back between the spaces of the bone just before the spinal cord, closer to the outside of your body. The needle is put in very slowly, and if you're wondering how the doctor knows he's in the right place, there's a very simple answer: the epidural space is full of air. Connected to the needle is a syringe full of air. When the doctor gets to the right space, the plunger of the needle depresses itself automatically. When this occurs, the doctor knows he may proceed. The needle is inserted into you extremely slowly, a millimeter at a time. All you will feel or sense is some pressure, nothing more. It should not hurt.

Once he gets into the epidural space, he'll put a catheter (a sterile plastic tube) into the needle, which is hollow. As he advances the catheter in through the needle, he will pass a few nerve fibers, and you may feel a sharp twinge in your buttocks. This will only last an instant, and the doctor will warn you of this feeling. When the catheter is in place, he'll take out the needle and tape the catheter to your back, up and over your shoulder. On the end of the catheter is an opening through which the doctor will inject the anesthesia. Thus, you won't feel relief during the procedure, which will take about fifteen to thirty minutes, but only after the anesthesia is injected into the catheter.

The doctor will inject a small amount of anesthetic at first, called the test dose, to see if you have any adverse reaction, such as an allergy. Five minutes later, he will administer the full dose. Within five to ten minutes you will begin to feel a warmth in your legs. You can still move your legs and wiggle your toes. There may be a tingling feeling before your legs get heavy or numb. But there will be no pain, and you will not feel the contractions. Slowly, they will be reduced to nothing more than an occasional sensation of pressure. Your nurse or coach may remark that on the monitor you're having a contraction, but by then you may be lying back with your eyes closed. "Who, me?" you'll reply.

The epidural does not take away sensations of temperature or pressure, but you cannot get out of bed and walk. There is a decrease in motor functioning. When you feel it wearing off, you can simply ask for some more, but do so right away. Epidurals can wear off rather quickly. They can last from forty-five minutes to three hours, depending on the strength of the dose administered.

When done properly, an epidural has no effect on the baby and is relatively safe for the mother, with no serious side effects. The mother will be awake during the birth, with her sensory perception and awareness unaffected. Epidurals can make birth a very pleasant experience.

On the other side, epidurals require that the woman's blood pressure be carefully monitored, as they do have a tendency, as mentioned, to cause blood pressure drops. Because a patient can have trouble pushing due to decreased sensation in the perineal and rectal areas, epidurals also increase the need for forceps deliveries. Forceps are safe, but, as in all areas of labor and delivery, the less intervention in the birth, the better. The anesthesia can be controlled so that it wears off in time to allow a woman to push, but most women having epidurals don't want to feel any more pain and do not take that option. Even if you are eager to push, you may find it difficult to return to full labor after the epidural wears off. The body builds up its own resistance to pain as it adjusts to the various levels of intensity; the pain at the end of labor might feel far worse.

Another disadvantage to the epidural is that it takes away the sensation in the bladder nerves, creating problems with urination. You won't feel the urge to urinate and your bladder will fill to capacity. During labor, a full bladder can prevent the baby's head from coming down. Catheterization may well be required to empty the bladder.

The postpartum pain for patients who have had epidurals can also be greater due to the more frequent use of forceps, because if forceps are required, you will have a bigger episiotomy and more stitches. Also, since your pain tolerance has not been built up throughout the labor, when the epidural wears off, everything will seem to hurt more. In addition to the extra need for forceps and catheters, an epidural may also require the patient to receive Pitocin, an artificial hormone, to augment what some doctors believe is a slowed-down labor with anesthesia. However, by not having an epidural too early you can make certain your labor is well established and there will be no need for Pitocin to stimulate it.

There are other anesthesias available. The most common—and the one freely given to most women—is a local anesthetic (frequently lidocaine) just for the episiotomy. Even in cases of natural childbirth they can be administered, and don't let anyone ever tell you that your childbirth wasn't natural if you've had this shot! It is given in the perineum at the time of delivery so that the cut of the episiotomy won't hurt. It will not change the way your contractions feel.

The pudendal block is given at the time of delivery as well. A longer needle, which blocks more than just the skin of the perineum as the local anesthetic does, is injected into the pudendal nerve. This is used for low forceps deliveries; it numbs more of your entire bottom.

Spinal anesthesia is injected into the cerebrospinal fluid in your lower back. It will make you numb from your waist to your feet. Women who are given spinal anesthesia are asked to lie flat for hours after delivery to help prevent the bad headaches that can occur from the anesthesia circulating in your head. Variations on the spinal can be given at different spots on the lower back, providing relief from the injection area downward. The popular saddle block of some years back, which is hardly used anymore, is one such procedure, but it blocks a smaller area than the spinal or the epidural. Spinals are almost never done; epidurals have taken their place. With all these choices of analgesics and anesthetics, how do you decide what is right for you and when you should use it?

Before you make any decision when you are in labor, remember the following points:

1. Don't make any decisions during a contraction. Make decisions only during the intervals in between. Some women will do and say anything during contractions.
2. Try switching your breathing. If you're doing slow chest, switch to shallow. If you're doing shallow, switch to one of the combined techniques. This may provide all the relief you need and put you back in control.
3. Change your position. A lot of your discomfort, particularly in back labor, can be alleviated by making your position more comfortable. Getting on all fours can help in back labor, for instance; sometimes the relief is immediate. The switch may get you through what is only a temporary loss of control.
4. Get yourself examined. Most doctors will do an examination before anesthesia is administered to make sure you're not nine centimeters and almost ready to deliver. But ask for an exam before you've made up your mind. It could be you're as slow as you imagine and some pain relief might be a blessing.

Memo to the Coach

This is one of the most important times for you to be supportive. Don't increase her guilt about having to ask for relief. Don't tell her she has to get through something that is very painful without any help. You're not going through the labor; she is.

How do you decide you might need anesthesia? This depends on how much you're losing control and how easily you think you can regain it. Remember that there are times during labor when it is natural to feel your energy flagging, to get depressed and exhausted, even paranoid and mistrustful. Your desire for anesthetic help may be linked to any one of these mood swings, so be aware of the cycles of labor. Go back to Chapter 10 and read over the mood changes that accompany each phase.

If you have decided that you absolutely must have something because you can no longer concentrate and do your breathing properly, because you have tried changing your position and you are exhausted from hours of labor, you have several choices. You can decide if you want complete pain relief for the rest of the labor or if you just want something to help you through a bad part. If you cannot decide this, the wisest thing to do would be to take the second step. Try an analgesic; ask for some Demerol. You can always have an epidural after the Demerol wears off, but having an epidural is a final decision.

We've been asked if we think that doctors and nurses affect your decision about anesthesia. It is certainly true that the presence of authority figures can alter a patient's desire, though we try not to tell people what to do. We simply recommend a course of action. The best thing you can do might be to ask the doctor and nurse to step out of the room while you make your decision. Talk it over with the coach and *do not* be pressured into anything you don't want. There are some doctors and nurses who push epidurals; they've seen a lot of women have very nice labors with anesthesia, and they don't want to see you suffer. Some doctors and nurses may not like anesthesia, and their presence may make you feel even guiltier. So decide on your own.

Remember that today, anesthesia is safe. If you need it, there's really no reason in the world not to have it. The ultimate goal, after all, is to have a healthy baby and a healthy mother, and as long as there are safe ways to relieve pain and you need that relief, you should use them. What seems silly to us is to see women coming in who are in very early labor, perhaps only one or two centimeters dilated, who ask for anesthesia immediately without even giving their labor a chance. They take anesthesia because they are afraid of what *might* happen, not because of what *is* happening.

There are also some people who come in afraid of epidurals because they think having a needle in their backs means they will end up paralyzed for life or with recurrent back problems or terrible headaches. There are times when you know that someone needs help, but when you offer it, the lack of knowledge becomes a terrible barrier. A sixteen-year-old boy brought his fifteen-year-old girl friend into the labor suite. She was scared to death and in terrible agony. She had taken no childbirth classes and had no idea what was happening to her. Seeing that she couldn't handle it, we tried to tell her about an epidural, because she needed complete pain relief by this time. It was explained that the epidural was not a spinal, that it did not cause headaches, or back trouble, or paralysis—and with this the boyfriend turned around and announced, "You're not putting anything into *her* back."

One of the nurses then took the young man aside. "Who are you to make any decision for her?" she said angrily. "If you had one contraction, I'm not sure you could be so brave. Give her a chance to listen. We don't do things to hurt people here. We do things to help them."

Sometimes women lose sight of their goal, that they're in labor to have a baby. You must always keep that in mind for it does help to make labor more bearable.

In the end, it is better to have a natural, spontaneous delivery than to have a low forceps delivery. It is better to go to the bathroom on your own than to be catheterized. Don't go to the hospital with the attitude that you want an epidural the second you walk in the door. Try the other things that have been suggested here first. Remember that even the most prepared people do fall apart when things go badly, and some women no one ever expected to go through with it have come in and made it from labor to delivery without any help at all. There's no way to predict what will happen to you.

The most important advice we can leave you with on the subject of anesthesia is to remain open and flexible, and not to make any decisions ahead of time. Don't say, I'll never have anything, no matter what. I want to do it with no help! Conversely, don't talk yourself into the kind of fear that leads to a total lack of confidence in your ability to handle things *without* help. No one is going to judge you for your decision—not your husband, not your doctor, not your nurse, and, especially, not your baby.

CHAPTER FIFTEEN

It Won't Happen to Me: Problems and Complications

One of the biggest problems in teaching prepared childbirth classes comes when the subject of problems and complications is broached. The immediate reaction of most of the women is to tune out what we are saying. This doesn't refer to me, they think. I'm not a breech. I'm not having any problems. I don't have diabetes. My baby is not too big. My blood pressure is low. The list of denials goes on and on. It's almost impossible to get most people to pay any attention at all.

The results of this attitude can be unfortunate. One woman from our classes came over to see us after the birth of her baby—by Cesarean section—and said, "I'm so upset with myself. You went into *everything* in class, but I really didn't believe it would be me, so I didn't pay any attention."

The moral of this story is, read this chapter and the following one on Cesareans carefully. *Don't* skip ahead to the chapter on postpartum; don't bury your head in the sand, believing that this information is all for "other people." Be prepared for anything that might happen. Pay attention. By the time you're in labor, you'll be in no mood to start learning; you'll be afraid if something out of the ordinary occurs, and your fear will make it worse. So here's your chance to be truly prepared.

When we speak of problems and complications, we're talking about alterations in the first and second stages of labor that make these labors different from the norm. This does not mean that there's anything seriously wrong; it simply means that these labors are not exactly the same as *textbook* labors. We're not speaking of lengthier phases. (For instance, if you're in active labor longer than the book says, that isn't a complication.) We're speaking of occurrences that change the course of your labor and delivery, even in some small way.

Remember that many so-called problems are really quite routine to doctors and nurses. Forceps deliveries fall into this category; fetal distress, with the advent of fetal monitors, can be just a minor thing that can be carefully observed. The same is true of meconium (see below) in the amniotic fluid. Many of the things we will be discussing happen often and usually end up perfectly normal.

While these changes in labor may be routine for the hospital staff, they are never routine for the patients. They always feel as if they're the only ones it has ever happened to. And you will feel the same way. By reading this chapter, and by understanding what is happening, you can help to alleviate much of this anxiety. And you will be one of the most truly prepared of expectant mothers. Have your coach read this material through as well, for often the anxiety of the woman's partner can make her feel worse. With both of you informed, the chances are you'll be able to face whatever happens feeling more confident in the face of any fears.

Ruptured Membranes

This subject has been discussed earlier, but since it can include some problems, it will be covered again here. The breaking of the membranes of your amniotic bag can occur prematurely—that is, they can rupture before labor begins. At that time the cervix may be thick and not ready for delivery. In approximately 90 percent of all cases, women will go into labor by themselves within twenty-four hours. Most doctors will not want to wait longer than that before inducing labor, so if your water bag breaks, you can be assured that within forty-eight hours, you'll deliver your baby.

If your water breaks before you're in labor, do not take any baths; do not have intercourse; do not put a tampon in your vagina. (If you're uncomfortably wet, put a maxi pad in your underwear.) You are more prone to infection without the protection of the amniotic fluid. Your doctor may want you to stay home and wait for your labor to begin, so conserve your energy. (Most doctors do want to be called when your water breaks, but ask your physician or midwife what the preferred procedure is. Some may not want to be informed if it's three in the morning.) There are some doctors who will be extra cautious and ask you to take your temperature every four hours to make sure there is no infection, as your vagina has microorganisms that can spread into the uterus and cause problems. If you are asked to take your temperature, don't be alarmed. It doesn't mean anything is wrong; it is simply a precautionary measure.

Your breaking water can cause a gush of fluid or a trickle, and it can be distinguished from urine because it is colorless and odorless. If you aren't sure if your water has broken, let your doctor take a look at you. If you do not go into labor within twenty-four hours, your doctor will probably want to induce labor. The subject of induction is covered later on in this chapter.

Meconium

Amniotic fluid is the water the baby floats in. As we have said before, it is colorless and odorless. The baby is constantly swallowing it when in utero. Sometimes when your water breaks, it has a color, which may be light yellow-green, brownish, or a darker green. This color means that the baby has passed meconium into the amniotic fluid. Meconium is the baby's first bowel movement, which is sterile and is a thick, tarlike substance. Most babies pass this within twenty-four hours of their birth. When it is passed in utero, it stains the fluid. The amount of meconium determines how thick and how colored the fluid is and can tell you how recently it was passed.

The presence of meconium usually indicates that the baby has been stressed at some point, and that its oxygen supply has been cut off temporarily. This should not alarm you, as it does not mean that the baby will have any physical problems as a result. It can mean that the baby has simply leaned on the cord, or that the cord was looped around its neck or one of its limbs, and that in moving, the cord was compressed for a moment and there was a temporary lack of oxygen. When this occurs, the anal sphincter muscle relaxes and the meconium is passed, which is basically a benign occurrence.

If the fluid is stained a light green, it means the meconium has been passed quite recently. Brownish fluid indicates older meconium. Often if a baby is postmature—that is, past its delivery date—there will be meconium in the fluid. If your water is stained at all, it's best to call your doctor right away. In most cases this amounts to absolutely nothing, but it can require closer surveillance and possibly induction, if your labor does not begin soon. Meconium is not a cause for panic, but it is not normal and your doctor might want to admit you to the hospital so you can be placed on a fetal monitor. The internal monitor will sometimes be used, since it is more accurate and more sensitive than the external monitor. The doctor will want to watch the baby simply to make certain the stress does not occur again. Once more, we're dealing with strictly precautionary measures. You will receive extra attention, but this does not mean there is something wrong with the baby, so don't worry. No one is assuming the baby is in trouble; they just want to make certain there is nothing to be worried about.

Induction

When labor is started artificially, it is called induction, and it is done by giving the woman a drug called Pitocin. Pitocin is a synthetic hormone, the generic name for which is oxytocin. Oxytocin is produced by the female body to stimulate labor. If the body does not produce the hormone in sufficient amounts either to start labor or to help it along enough, the woman may be given Pitocin to supplement her body's own levels. Pitocin and oxytocin have only one function: they work on the pregnant uterus. They have no effect on a nonpregnant woman or on a man.

Since it is extremely potent, Pitocin is given intravenously in very controlled amounts. The treatment needs careful monitoring, for only minuscule amounts are required to get the needed effect. It can be dangerous if overused, so a nurse will be present at all times if you get Pitocin. Pitocin will have an effect similar to that of oxytocin on your labor—that is, your labor will start slowly and gradually build up and get stronger—but it works much faster. In fact, it can cut the duration of a labor in half.

Pitocin is given to induce a labor, to start it off from point zero, or to augment a labor, and to speed up a slow labor already in progress. It is also given after delivery to help your uterus contract to its normal size, either intramuscularly or intravenously.

There are many reasons for induction. Premature rupture of membranes, discussed earlier in this chapter, is one. Another is if you are two weeks overdue. The reason for this is that the placenta does not function as well after forty-two weeks, and the baby can be deprived of essential nutrients and oxygen. Most doctors will not allow a pregnancy to last longer than forty-two weeks.

Medical problems are another reason for induction. If you suffer from diabetes, toxemia, hypertension, or other conditions that will be exacerbated by the stress and strain of pregnancy, your doctor may want to induce labor before your due date.

Remember that induction is not done for reasons of convenience. (For instance, your doctor will not induce you simply because you want the baby born on your wedding anniversary.) Induction is not the preferred method of delivering a baby. Your own oxytocin results in a more gradual labor that is less stressful to the baby. Induced labor causes harder contractions and much more powerful uterine activity. That is why a nurse is always present. She will watch the heartbeat of the baby and monitor the duration, frequency, and intensity of your contractions to make sure you're not being given too much of the drug.

Most people who are induced—that is, those who have their labors started artificially from scratch—have epidurals. The labor becomes quite intense and very hard. It can also take some time to get it started, since the induced cervix is usually an uneffaced, unripened cervix. This can lead to two-day inductions, or even Cesareans if the induction does not work. Pitocin can cut the time of dilatation of the cervix in half, but it does not cut effacement time. If the induction doesn't work, you may get sent home to wait until it is tried again the next day.

A side effect of Pitocin is that it can cause overstimulation of the uterus. The problem here is that the uterus doesn't relax properly between contractions, so the baby's heartbeat may slow down. If the contractions last too long, they can affect the proper flow of blood to the baby. But the drug is administered very carefully and regulated closely so that it can be increased or decreased immediately. And Pitocin has a very short half-life; if the flow gets shut off, it stops working right away. Within five minutes, you should feel the contractions slow and stop.

Augmentation

Pitocin is also used to stimulate sluggish labors. The reason for this is that labor is a very stressful event for both the baby and the mother and there are limits to the strength and endurance of both. If it's obvious that a labor isn't progressing very well, augmenting the labor may be necessary. The doctor or nurse can tell if a labor is not progressing by examinations. In the active phase, on the average, a woman will dilate one centimeter every hour once she reaches four centimeters. If you are not progressing properly—if you're four centimeters at 9:00 A.M. and by 1:00 P.M. you're only five centimeters—you may need some help. In a case like this, you might or might not be contracting. You may be having one contraction every ten minutes, or one every three minutes. The pains may feel very strong but they might not be strong enough to help the labor progress. If the contractions are not effective, your labor may have to be augmented, especially if you have high blood pressure or some other medical problem.

Augmentation is handled the same way as induction, with the Pitocin administered in an I.V. and monitored by a nurse. But it is different from induction in that the woman is already in labor and has begun to dilate. The Pitocin will work quickly to speed up the labor and will not necessarily result in the need for an epidural. Pitocin can be administered at any point in the labor, including right up to the time of delivery. And the speed with which you will notice the Pitocin taking effect is quite different. In an induction it can take an hour before a woman really notices the contractions, which may have begun within fifteen minutes of administering the drug. In augmentation, you will notice a building up in intensity within five minutes.

The two biggest fears about Pitocin, which has become a kind of dirty word to some natural childbirth advocates, are that it is given arbitrarily and that it will cause agony the minute it is administered. Neither of these is true. The contractions will build up gradually, just as in a normal labor, and will *not* result in an immediate wall of pain. And Pitocin is not given for the doctor's convenience. It is given only for reasons of medical necessity.

Fetal Distress

Another problem that has become more common now that mothers are routinely monitored in labor is fetal distress. There are times when the baby's heartbeat may slow down, and this can be heard on the fetal monitor. When the heartbeat goes more slowly, there are reasons, but they are not—again—necessarily serious. They are simply a cause for careful observation.

Most of the time, a decrease in the rate of the baby's heartbeat indicates some oxygen deprivation. This *does not* mean brain damage. The heartbeat goes down reflexively in response to several conditions:

1. The head may be compressed. This is a sign that the baby's head is moving down, a good sign that you are getting closer to full dilatation. This decrease in heartbeat is usually associated with the peak of the contraction. Unless labor is unduly prolonged at this point, nothing needs to be done.

2. The cord may be compressed. If the baby is leaning on the cord or if the cord is wrapped around its neck or around a limb, the heartbeat may drop in response to the compression. Changing your position may alleviate this problem.

3. The placenta is not giving the baby enough oxygen. You may be given an oxygen mask to help give you and your baby more oxygen.

In addition to changing your position, putting on an

oxygen mask, and elevating your feet (to take pressure off your pelvis), you may have an internal monitor placed inside you if you don't already have one. You may also be turned onto your left side to get the weight of the uterus off the major vessels leading into the right side of the heart. This positioning will lead to improved circulation that increases the oxygen flow to your baby. Your I.V. fluids may be increased, and you will be examined. This flurry of activity may make you nervous, but remember that it is only being done to make certain nothing is wrong. It does not mean that there *is* something wrong.

Years ago, many instances of fetal distress went unnoticed due to the fact that fetal monitors were not in common use. Nowadays, problems with deliveries can be avoided by monitoring. For example, a baby exhibiting fetal distress can be tested quite simply to see if it is getting enough oxygen. A fetal scalp Ph is done—the baby's head is pricked slightly to draw a drop of blood, which is then tested in a machine to see what the oxygen level in that blood is. The technique, unavailable until recently, can let the woman know that the baby is okay.

Forceps Delivery

The use of forceps, which has been mentioned in connection with epidural anesthesia, is also considered part of a labor that deviates from the norm. Forceps look like two spoons with the centers cut out that are separate but hook together on the handles, below the spoon-shaped part. Each side of the forceps (the spoon shape) fits over the side of the baby's head; forceps *never* go over the face. They cover an area of the head from the top to just below the ear. They are used during the second stage of labor when a woman is having difficulty pushing out the baby on her own. This may be caused by an epidural, which makes it harder to push correctly due to lack of sensation, or the way a woman's body is constructed, or the size of the baby being born. Two hours of pushing is usually the maximum a doctor will allow, due to the stress on the baby. Forceps may then be used to help with the delivery. (The baby's head must be low enough for forceps to be considered safe. If this is not the case, forceps will not be used and a Cesarean may be necessary.)

Forceps are not dangerous to the baby when they are properly used. They can cause some bruising—usually marks on either side of the head or face near the ears—but this commonly disappears within twenty-four hours. Some hospitals use vacuum aspirators instead of forceps. A cone is placed on the baby's head and the baby is pulled out by force of suction. Since the vacuum aspirator is relatively new and requires special training for its use, many doctors prefer forceps, with which they are more familiar.

Forceps are very helpful and can assist you in delivering a very healthy baby. When they are used, you usually will be given anesthesia; if you haven't had an epidural, you will most likely be given a pudendal block.

There is no reason to feel guilty if you have a forceps delivery. It does not necessarily mean that you haven't pushed correctly. Sometimes your baby will simply need just a little bit of help to get over the pelvic arch, and this is what the forceps provide.

Multiple Births

Multiple births can bring complications of their own. If you are carrying twins or triplets (or more), you will most likely know it ahead of time, and your doctor will explain everything you need to know. But if you are carrying more than one child, there are a few things about labor you should keep in mind. One is, when you go into labor don't stay at home. Your pregnancy has been followed more carefully than that of a woman with one fetus, and your labor and delivery will be more carefully monitored as well. Go right to the hospital. The labors of women with multiple fetuses normally go more slowly because the larger bulk of the uterus doesn't contract as well, but many multiple births are premature or a bit early because of this extra weight pressing down. With twins, problems of labor and delivery depend on the position of the babies. Usually, when you come to the hospital in labor both of your babies will be monitored, one at a time. An internal monitor will be used on one, an external on the other. And there's one thing you can depend on with a multiple birth: you are sure to have an audience. There will be pediatricians, an anesthesiologist on standby, several nurses to take care of the babies, medical students, nursing students, and anyone else around who wants to watch. Don't be disconcerted by all these people. It can make the births very exciting. If it does bother you, though, you have the right to ask all but the doctors and the nurses to leave.

Babies born of multiple births tend to be smaller than the average, and there are no set rules as to what will occur at the time of their births: you cannot depend on having two vaginal births if you have twins, since this will depend entirely on the position of the babies when you go into labor. If your first baby is born head down, it may be delivered vaginally and the second delivered breech (see below) or with forceps. A breech position for the first baby almost always dictates a Cesarean section. Your doctor will explain the various positions of the babies to you in advance and will tell you what his preferred method of delivery is.

Postmature Babies

Two common deviations from average birth experiences are premature and postmature babies. Postmature babies are defined as babies that have gone "full term"—have been in utero forty-two weeks or more. Sometimes you may be late delivering, up to two weeks in fact, but by strict definition you are only "late"; you are not postmature. But anyone who has passed her delivery date can expect her doctor to watch her carefully, and possibly to ask her to take a nonstress test. This test requires you to be hooked up to an external monitor, as described in Chapter 12, and to press a button whenever you feel the baby move. The baby's heartbeat is correlated with its movements, to see if the heartbeat increases with the movements.

After forty-two weeks pass, the placenta does not function as well as it has throughout the pregnancy. It begins, little by little, to deteriorate, and it doesn't transport nutrients and oxygen as well as it did. The baby has to be watched more closely. If you pass forty-two weeks, your doctor may try induction, but if your cervix is not ready and has not yet "ripened," your chances of a Cesarean section increase.

Postmature and even simply overdue babies often look bigger than term babies, since they have gained more weight. Their skin may be peeling, due to dryness, since the protective vernix that nature provides for the baby in the amniotic fluid has worn off. They may be wrinkled due to longer immersion in the fluid, and they may even look older. Some may have passed meconium inside the uterus.

Premature Babies

Those babies who are born at thirty-seven weeks or earlier or who are under five pounds at birth, even if they are full term, are defined as premature. After birth, these babies are immediately sent to the intensive care unit, where they are given careful monitoring and supervision to make certain there are no problems.

If you go into premature labor after your water has broken, most of the time no attempt will be made to stop the labor, since the barrier to infection is no longer there. If your water hasn't broken, the doctors and nurses will try to stop your labor. In recent years, they've had more success because of the introduction of new drugs.

Years ago, if a woman went into premature labor, there were not many ways it could be halted. Alcohol came to be a popular way to stop labor—not in the form of a glass of wine but rather given intravenously. Women given alcohol through an I.V. got very, very drunk, and their labors sometimes stopped, because the uterus is a muscle and alcohol is a muscle relaxant. If the uterus is contracted, it is in an unrelaxed state. After trying alcohol, hospitals switched to an antihypertensive called Hyperstat, but that had severe side effects because it caused a drop in blood pressure. Today, a new drug called Ritodrine works extremely well. It is given intravenously and works almost immediately to stop the contractions.

If you are in premature labor, get to the hospital at once. The faster you come in, the more that can be done to help you. Remember that there is a difference between premature contractions, which you may feel but which aren't doing anything to change your cervix, and premature labor, in which your cervix has begun to efface and dilate. Labor can be stopped even if a woman is dilated five centimeters.

Of course, not all premature labors should be stopped. For instance, if a baby is not growing properly in utero, it would be better to have that baby prematurely, even if the baby is smaller and younger. In this case, the concern is lung development rather than size. If it is determined that the baby will have a good chance to breathe on its own, the labor will not be interrupted if something is wrong with the pregnancy.

If the labor is to be stopped, the woman is given Ritodrine intravenously and put to bed. She is kept in the hospital on an I.V. for twenty-four hours and is carefully monitored. She is then given Ritodrine pills every two hours for twenty-four hours, and following that, her dosage is slowly tapered. She may be on Ritodrine for the rest of her pregnancy.

Ritodrine has no side effects on the baby that have been recognized as yet, but there are side effects on the mother. It can cause severe tachycardia (racing of the heart), it can make the woman jittery and very nervous, and it can lower potassium levels. The baby's heartbeat may increase as well.

Usually the doctor will stop Ritodrine at thirty-six weeks to see whether the woman will go into labor by herself or not. A baby born then is considered virtually full term.

Premature babies, born of labors that cannot be stopped, are much smaller than normal. A baby born at twenty-seven to twenty-eight weeks is considered viable, and steroids can now be administered to speed up lung development in the fetus. The baby will look comparatively scrawny and skinny because it will not have the layer of fat under its skin that develops during the last few weeks in utero. Premature babies also seem very frail and fragile. The baby will be placed in the intensive care unit, which may be a very scary experience for the mother and father. But it is important for you to feel reassured by this, for the baby is getting the care it needs. Talk to the pediatricians and feel free to ask all the questions you want.

And remember that premature labor does not necessarily mean there is something wrong with the baby. In some cases, it can be caused by structural anomalies in the mother—if her cervix, for instance, cannot support the pressure of a growing fetus. However, there may still be problems with the baby when it is born, due to its prematurity.

Breech Delivery

This last problem to be discussed will be covered more extensively in the next chapter on Cesareans. Breech position means that the feet or buttocks are being born first, which complicates the delivery of the baby. If it is your first baby, most doctors will do a Cesarean section; if you've never had a child before, there's no way a doctor can be certain that the head will fit. (The baby's head is the largest part of its body. Born head first, the rest fits. Born feet first, the baby might get stuck if the head is large.) But if your doctor has determined that the baby is small or that it does not have an unusually large head (sometimes an X ray can show this), you may still be able to deliver vaginally with the breech position. You will not be given an epidural, because pushing is very, very important in this case. You will be considered a high-risk delivery and your labor will be monitored more closely. If your doctor has determined ahead of time that your baby is breech, go to the hospital as soon as your labor begins, or as soon as the water breaks.

All of these various problems and complications can be troubling, especially when they're grouped together like this. Try to remember that perhaps only one or none of these things may happen to you; it's highly unlikely all of them will. And remember, too, that when you're in labor, it's okay to be scared if something unexpected happens. You're going to feel that you're the only person in the world that this has ever happened to; that everything your friends told you about labor and delivery is wrong; that something is wrong with your baby. But that is why you are in a hospital, a facility prepared to handle these problems.

Knowing what's happening to you can make all of this easier to bear. Not everything is as horrendous as it may seem; there are a lot of things that will be done as a matter of course. All of the monitoring that's necessary, for instance, does not indicate that the baby is in trouble. Ask questions if you're not sure what's happening to you. Many times doctors and nurses may be quite busy, moving in a big hurry all around you and unable to answer your questions right away. But we'll give you an answer after the commotion has quieted down. Then you can find out what was done and why we did it.

Find out if there is any cause for concern. Your doctor and nurses will be honest with you and they will tell you. No one is trying to keep anything from you, because we need your cooperation, too. Perhaps in the old days the attitude was, Don't let her know, but that is no longer true. We don't hide anything. We're there to help you and to keep you informed. *You* and your baby are our prime concern.

CHAPTER SIXTEEN

Surgery Without Guilt: The Cesarean Section

In an era when there are very sophisticated ways to determine if there are problems with a pregnancy, many doctors would rather be safe and perform a Cesarean section than leave anything to chance. Statistics indicate that one out of five babies is delivered abdominally, with anesthesia, rather than vaginally. And with this in mind, you are strongly advised to read this chapter, even though most women prefer *not* to think about this possibility.

In our classes we can tell what's going on in the mothers' minds: Ho hum, this won't happen to me. I really don't want to hear about it. And besides, it scares me! And they half-listen and half-block out everything we say.

Over and over we tell them, "Listen. This could be the most important thing you learn about."

Are you listening?

Planning for the possibility of a Cesarean section can work just like prepared childbirth or any other technique. By learning what to expect, you can make the experience a better one. By being informed and relaxed, you can decrease the amount of pain and discomfort following surgery. A difference in your attitude is all you need. Even with a Cesarean section, you can help yourself. Cesareans are scary, we admit, but if you know what will happen, you'll approach the procedure with far more calm and confidence.

It's easy to deny the need for any knowledge of this procedure; many women do not know ahead of time that they will have to have one. In fact, for the majority of people having their first babies, a Cesarean is unplanned.

The biggest cause of the rise in the Cesarean section rate is the advancement in fetal monitoring and fetal diagnostic techniques. Years ago, these options were not available and many complications went undetected, resulting in problem babies and difficult births. Now doctors can discover these problems; they can be detected when the woman is in labor, or even ahead of time, with sonography (the use of ultrasound waves to produce an image of the unborn child). Breech presentations and fetal anomalies can be discovered in advance of birth. The fetal heart monitor, unheard of years ago, is now routine in most hospitals. The fetal heart rate is monitored throughout the active phase and changes in its patterns can be detected and analyzed.

Another reason for the higher Cesarean rate is the more advanced age of women giving birth. Doctors consider many women over thirty in the high-risk category because advanced maternal age can lead to more complicated deliveries. Their pregnancies and labors are monitored more closely.

Many women are also giving birth to fewer babies; a drop in the birth rate per couple means that each one born is more of a "premium baby" and is treated as more precious cargo. Methods of delivery that may have caused problems in the past, such as high forceps, are no longer used. A lower-risk Cesarean is done instead.

It is interesting to note that as the Cesarean section rate has gone up, the maternal morbidity and infant mortality rates have declined (mortality means death; morbidity refers to problems resulting from injury or damage). In fact, of all abdominal surgery, Cesarean section has the lowest mortality and morbidity rate. It is considered to be major abdominal surgery, but its success has to do, in part, with the fact that the patients are mainly healthy young women. The risks of the surgery are so low that it is not considered to be a risk to the mother. In the past, there used to be complications resulting from Cesareans, and the procedure was not taken lightly.

The main problem with Cesareans is psychological—many women believe that having a baby vaginally makes them in some way superior. This attitude leads to a great deal of guilt when a delivery through the pelvis is not possible. In fact, attitude can play a large role in Cesarean birth, and by being educated about the procedure, you can make it a lot easier on yourself should you turn out to be one of the one in five who has a "section."

That advice is not as easy to follow as it may seem. Information to help you prepare for Cesarean section is not widely available. First of all, most women have no idea they're going to need a Cesarean. There are several books available, but you may not want to buy a book if you feel all is going well with your pregnancy. Second, although there are many childbirth preparation classes available, many spend little or no time at all on the possible complications of pregnancy and delivery; the result is that more women are completely unprepared.

When you do try to become informed, you'll find that Cesareans have a terrible public image. They are thought by many to be overused, dangerous, disfiguring surgery that should be avoided at all costs. You are now aware that their use is tied to diagnostic techniques and that their danger is at a minimum. What about vanity? If long, puckered Cesarean scars frighten you, remember that many doctors prefer the neater incision known as the bikini cut, a low, horizontal incision that heals neatly and can be easily hidden by the bathing suit for which it is named. The vertical incision is still used in emergencies, as it is by far the faster of the two.

Finally, women are afraid that having one Cesarean means that any baby they have in the future must be delivered by Cesarean. This will depend on the type of uterine incision you've had, your doctor's practices, and the reason for the first Cesarean section. If you have had a vertical incision into your uterus, you will most likely have to have another Cesarean, since the incision in your uterus is at the top (the fundus), where contractions are felt the hardest and the scar is most likely to rupture. You will be scheduled for your second Cesarean a week or two before your due date, so as to avoid any possibility that you might go into labor. If you have had a horizontal incision into your uterus—known as a low flap incision—your uterus will have a scar on its lowest part, which absorbs the least amount of pressure during a contraction. The fear that the scar will rupture is considerably diminished. You will be allowed a trial of labor provided all goes well. A vaginal delivery following an initial Cesarean section is determined to a large extent by a woman's willingness to have one. Wanting it badly enough may really help. You will not, however, be allowed to remain in labor if the labor does not progress normally, as Pitocin will not be given to you.

The reasons for your first Cesarean will affect your second birth as well. If the first Cesarean was done because the baby's head was too big, chances are the second baby will be just as big or even bigger, so you'll probably have another Cesarean. If your problem was herpes, the disease could activate again. But if your first delivery was affected by malpresentation, abruption (see below), placenta previa (see below), or some kind of fetal distress, it is entirely possible that your second birth will be perfectly normal and a vaginal delivery may be possible. Talk over your feelings with your doctor. The old idea of once a C section, always a C section, is starting to give way.

Cesareans got their bad name partly by the manner in which they were performed. In many hospitals, patients were taken off the labor floor up to an operating room to have their surgery, thus isolating and stigmatizing the patient at the start. General anesthesia was commonly used, so the mother missed the entire birth experience and never got to see or hold her baby until well after surgery was finished. Fathers were never allowed in the operating room, and in general the atmosphere of birth was exchanged for one of surgery.

Today, there are many hospitals in which the delivery room on the labor floor is also used as the operating room. Epidural anesthesia can be used for many Cesareans, so that the mother can be awake and aware during delivery and can hold and nurse her baby following its birth. There is a new movement toward allowing fathers into the operating room, but only in those cases in which there is some advance warning of surgery. In all, hospitals are now trying to make the Cesarean birth more of a *birth* experience.

One of the problems with Cesarean section is that in the case of nonelective, or emergency, Cesareans, there is no time to prepare psychologically for what is about to happen. In cases of real fetal distress, there is a "rush back" emergency in which no one has time to explain anything. In these cases, even preparation may not help with the difficulty and fright caused by the emergency. Not only is the mother worried about the threat to her of the unplanned surgery she is facing, she is panicked over the fate of her baby.

When a Cesarean is planned, the attitude can be very different. A doctor may know ahead of time that your baby is going to be a breech delivery, and he may recommend a Cesarean because the baby is large. If you have herpes, placenta previa (a condition in which the placenta may cover the cervical opening), diabetes, or toxemia, you may know in advance that you will have surgery. Even if these things are noted when you are in the hospital, in labor, you can be prepared.

But remember, you may not have any choice about what happens. Cesareans are doctors' decisions. The major reasons for a Cesarean section include the following:

Cephalopelvic Disproportion

This situation is usually discovered when you are in labor. It means that the baby's head may be larger than your pelvic opening. It does not necessarily mean that the baby is huge—only that there is some reason why the progression of labor has stopped and the baby's head has not descended properly. If the cervix has stopped dilating, the doctors will almost always give you some Pitocin to stimulate your uterus and make sure it's not inadequate contractions that are causing the lack of progress. If that does not work after a reasonable amount of time, you will have a Cesarean section.

The doctor will have some definite clues ahead of time that this condition exists. For instance, if the cervix remains thick and uneffaced and the baby's head is riding high and doesn't engage before the woman goes into labor, it may be because the head is too large for the opening. A woman having her first baby should engage two weeks before delivery; if the head is not engaged when labor starts, it probably will not engage at all. By the time you're fully dilated, the head *should* be at zero station, which means the baby is descending properly. But with cephalopelvic disproportion you probably will never be fully dilated, because it is the direct pressure of the baby's head on the cervix that causes dilatation. Years ago, doctors tried a mid or high forceps in some of these cases, and at times this did result in damage to the baby.

Breech Birth

Breech is the most common form of what is called *malpresentation,* when the baby is not presenting head down, as is common, but feet first, bottom first, or sometimes just lying across your uterus horizontally (transverse). Since the head is the largest part of the baby, the body can slip through the pelvis easily, but no one wants to risk not knowing the size of the head. If you have had more than one baby, then the doctor has some idea what size your pelvis is; with your first baby, he doesn't, and therefore he will want to do a Cesarean section in case there is cephalopelvic disproportion.

Placenta Previa

This condition is usually noticed prior to the onset of labor. It occurs when the placenta grows either partially or completely over the opening of the cervix rather than being attached to the side or the top of the uterus. This can cause bleeding (painless and bright red) in the third trimester as the cervix changes and softens, and the bleeding can enable the doctor to diagnose the condition. It is also easily diagnosed through sonography. You will then have a Cesarean section. Since there is a difference between a low-lying placenta and a placenta previa, you may require an examination when you are in the hospital. In this case, you will be examined right in the operating room. Should there be a placenta previa, a Cesarean will be performed immediately. A low-lying placenta can also cause bleeding, but it is not necessarily a reason for a Cesarean.

Herpes

If you have *herpes genitalia,* this poses no serious threat or harm to you, but it does pose an extremely serious threat to the baby. If your herpes is active and you have a vaginal delivery, the baby will pass through an actively infected area, and this may lead to death or brain damage. Since the stress of pregnancy can lead to the activation of herpes, your doctor will test you regularly to make certain yours is not active. On the basis of these test results and how close you are to delivery, he will decide whether to perform a Cesarean. If your herpes is active and your water breaks, you must have a Cesarean within a few hours, as the infection can travel up to the baby once the barrier of the amniotic fluid is gone. If you suffer from herpes, you should check with your doctor as to what rules your hospital nursery has about babies of mothers with herpes. In some hospitals, you may not touch your newborn baby; if you do, the baby must then stay with you in your room at all times. It will not be allowed back in the nursery with the other babies. In this case, you will be "rooming-in" with your baby. After a Cesarean this can be difficult, so speak with your doctor in advance about what choices are available.

Fetal Distress

Fetal distress that is not an emergency was discussed in the last chapter. When it is clear that the problems with monitoring the baby's heart may mean further complications, a Cesarean can result. If the heartbeat slows and does not come back up and the doctor is not sure why, he may perform a Cesarean at once. Another reason for an emergency C section related to fetal distress occurs in the very rare case of a prolapsed cord. This is a condition in which the umbilical cord slips through the cervix before the baby's head. The main cause is the rupture of membranes when the head is unengaged. If the baby's head is so high up or the baby is in breech position and there is a good deal of space around the opening of the cervix, the force of the fluid rushing down from the broken water bag pushes the umbilical cord through the cervix. This is a real emergency, since the baby's head pushing down on top of the cord can compress it and shut off the baby's oxygen. The doctor will hold the baby's head off the cord until another physician performs a Cesarean section to lift the baby out.

Abruption

This is a condition in which the placenta either partially or completely peels away from the uterine wall. It usually starts during labor and can be recognized when the woman experiences contractions with no letup in pain. There is bleeding associated with abruptions, but it can be what is known as silent bleeding, in which the blood collects in pools behind the placenta. It is also usually associated with fetal distress. Early in the pregnancy, an abruption can cause a miscarriage, and later on it can lead to a stillbirth. But when it occurs in the third trimester, there is bleeding associated with it. The woman may bleed visibly, or the amniotic fluid can be bloody. An emergency Cesarean section follows the discovery of the condition.

Failure to Progress

If your labor does not result in the dilatation of your cervix, if it changes extremely slowly or not at all, you will then be induced. In some cases, induction will fail because the cervix is too thick and uneffaced, and in those cases, a Cesarean section will then be performed. Sometimes the reason for the lack of progression is cephalopelvic disproportion; other times the cause can be membranes that have ruptured before the cervix is ready. If you are two centimeters dilated for hours, and still two or three after you are induced, you may have to have a C section.

Medical Reasons

Conditions such as diabetes, toxemia (also known as preeclampsia), and other such medical complications in their severest forms can lead to Cesarean sections. Preeclampsia is a complication of pregnancy that can occur in mild to severe cases. Your blood pressure increases, you will suffer from edema (retention of fluids), protein will be present in your urine, and you may be hyperreflexive (your leg jerks excessively when the doctor taps your knee with a rubber hammer). The only cure for this disease is delivery. If the mother is suffering from such a disease, or from a medical problem such as diabetes (which can be exacerbated or caused by pregnancy), a Cesarean section can be performed ahead of the delivery date. The diseases of pregnancy, such as toxemia, will reverse themselves. Preexisting diseases will improve. In earlier days, it was generally believed that cardiac patients had to undergo Cesareans, but today, with epidurals administered during the second stage, they can have vaginal deliveries.

What happens to you during a Cesarean section?

In a nonemergency situation, when the Cesarean is either planned or there is adequate time, an epidural is administered. (Generally, with a planned Cesarean, you have been in the hospital for a day.) If a Cesarean is decided on and you have already had an epidural, you are given a larger dose of anesthesia sufficient for a Cesarean. If you have not had an epidural and there is time, you are given one.

In a nonemergency Cesarean, the nurse will probably shave your abdomen and part of your pubic hair. Some nurses shave everything (full prep). A Foley catheter will be inserted into your bladder to drain your urine throughout the surgery.

Your husband may be permitted in the delivery room. Ask your doctor if this is possible.

Once the epidural has taken effect, or if you're having general anesthesia, you are wheeled back to the operating room. As mentioned, this could be a regular operating room in another part of the hospital, or it could be one of the delivery rooms right on the labor floor. As you are wheeled in, the doctors and nurses will be scrubbing up and gloving and gowning, as this is a sterile surgical procedure. You will be transferred to the operating table. The anesthesiologist is usually your best friend during a Cesarean; he will be right at your head and will talk to you during the procedure. Most anesthesiologists will give you some oxygen with a mask before the surgery. The extra oxygen will give the baby a boost before it's born. Your own doctor will be present as well as another doctor or resident (if it's a teaching hospital) to assist during surgery. In addition, there will be a scrub nurse, a circulating nurse, and, in many hospitals, a pediatrician.

The doctors will put on their caps and gowns and then they will begin. They will wash your belly with Betadine and place sterile drapes on you. The anesthesiologist will also place a screen between you and your belly so you will not see the actual surgery taking place. A nurse will bring over the operating room table with the instruments, and the doctor will say, "Ready." If you are having general anesthesia, this is the time at which you will be put to sleep. They wait as long as possible, because the general anesthesia will reach the baby within five to ten minutes, so the very last thing they do before cutting is to knock you out.

During general anesthesia, which is administered intravenously and is probably sodium pentathol or a similar anesthetic, the anesthesiologist will stick a tube down your throat so you can breathe during the surgery. Some women wake up with sore throats from this procedure.

Surgery begins. The doctor cuts through the skin and into the uterus. The baby is born within five to ten minutes. (The rest of the hour that the Cesarean normally takes is used to repair the uterus and skin with stitches or staples.) The doctor lifts the baby up and out by placing a hand in your uterus; the assistant applies pressure to your fundus (the top of your uterus), and the baby is lifted up. Some babies cry immediately, even before they've been lifted up. They come out looking rather nice, with rounded heads and few bruises if you have not been in labor. But since they have not experienced the squeezing of the birth canal, which helps to clear their lungs, they may be slower to begin their respiration (which is why a vaginal delivery is preferable).

Cesarean babies are placed in isolettes, small glass boxes, in which they are kept for twenty-four hours in the nursery while they are carefully watched.

Your incision, which is almost always horizontal unless your surgery was an emergency (in which case the doctor makes a vertical cut), is stitched up or stapled and you will then be sent to the recovery room for several hours (this time varies from hospital to hospital). One reason why the epidural is the preferred anesthesia for a Cesarean is that you will be left relatively pain-free for one to two hours after surgery. When you wake up from general anesthesia, you feel pain right away.

Pitocin will be given to you intravenously to help your uterus contract, and if you have been in labor a long time before your eventual surgery, you might also be given antibiotics to prevent infection. If all goes well with your Cesarean section, it can be a very nice experience.

Some of the problems with Cesareans can occur postoperatively. You'll be fed intravenously for one or two days instead of having the I.V. taken out immediately, as happens following a vaginal birth. And you will be in the hospital longer, as long as seven days as opposed to three or four. There are problems with gas following the surgery and, of course, there's the pain of the incision and stitches.

There are things you can do to help ease these problems. You can be made more comfortable with your surgery by doing deep breathing exercises and by coughing, no matter how much these things hurt. It's important to expand your lungs, which promotes recovery and healing. Move from side to side and get up out of bed and walk. To make your stitches feel better, try taking a pillow, placing it over your abdomen, holding it there, and breathing deeply. The best thing of all is to get moving as soon as possible.

It's also important for you to find a comfortable position for breast-feeding, if that is what you have chosen for you and your baby. Some positions will be better than others. Don't feel you have to rush to get the baby to your breast; first make sure you are feeling all right about yourself. And don't be afraid to ask for pain medication! Most women hesitate because if they're nursing, they're afraid it's going to get into the baby. Medication will pass into your breast milk, but in such minuscule amounts that you have no reason to worry. It is better for the baby that you be comfortable and relaxed during nursing than uncomfortable and unhappy with pain.

Your Foley catheter may also make you feel uncomfortable, but that will be removed after twenty-four hours. Most women are told to get out of bed the next day following surgery. Don't be afraid to follow the nurse's instructions and to get up and walk. You won't tear anything or hurt yourself by moving around.

On the plus side, there are a few things Cesarean mothers don't have to go through that women do experience after vaginal deliveries. Take comfort in the fact that you don't have golf-ball-sized hemorrhoids from pushing at the end of labor; that your vaginal canal is not stretched out after a seven- or eight-pound baby has passed through; and that you have no episiotomy stitches to itch and cause you pain. As with vaginal deliveries, wait until your first postpartum doctor visit for permission to resume sexual relations.

Your attitude about Cesareans may be the most important factor of all. The ultimate goal, as we have so often said, is to have a healthy mother and a healthy baby. In terms of the entire outcome, the process itself is really of little importance. The surgery will not hurt you permanently, and you will recover faster than you think. In fact, no one will be able to tell that you had a Cesarean. You'll look the same as every other mother. And the important thing is that you should *feel* the same, too. Your delivery was something you did to ensure the health and well-being of your baby.

CHAPTER SEVENTEEN

Thank Goodness That's Over: The Recovery Room

Everyone expects to feel very "high" following the birth of the baby. It's natural to imagine a rosy glow over everything, to fantasize a beautiful pink and white (or blue and white) scene of smiling mother, placid newborn, everything natural and in complete harmony.

It's a surprise, then, to discover that sometimes your feelings following the baby's birth may not be all that you expected. For one thing, the baby that is handed to you may be far different from the baby you imagined. Your real baby may be screaming, its head may be misshapen from the journey through the birth canal, or its face may be bruised or marked by forceps. In addition, it may be the "wrong" sex or may not look like you or your husband. You may have strange feelings of not recognizing this tiny person.

In addition, you may be surprised by the sharp changes in your mood after the baby's birth. Throughout your pregnancy and especially during the last few months, you have been cushioned by a variety of hormones that have made you feel peaceful and serene. Nature provides for pregnant women in many ways, emotions included. When the baby is born, the hormones start to change and you may be left feeling less than secure and far from in control.

It's all right to have feelings of doubt or worry after you give birth. Don't be ashamed. You're not the first person to feel that way! By understanding the physical and emotional aspects of your postpartum condition, you can help yourself, both by knowing what to expect and what to do and by allowing yourself to express your feelings. Keeping everything bottled up inside will only make it worse.

Your first stop after delivery is probably the recovery room. Some hospitals take you straight to your own room; others require longer or shorter periods in the recovery room itself.

The baby will come into the recovery room with you for the first ten or fifteen minutes. This is an ideal time to breast-feed the baby or at least to try to begin breast-feeding. Some babies simply won't be interested, so don't be worried if yours doesn't start so soon after birth. But in the quiet of the recovery room you'll have time to get to know your baby a bit. Fathers should stay with the mother and baby for these first minutes, because it is at this time that all three begin the important process of *bonding*, of becoming a family. The closeness of the family unit at the start can lead to better feeling in the future. Get to know your baby: you can start right away.

We are familiar with the policy of keeping mothers who've delivered vaginally in the recovery room for two hours. You will be observed and checked often by a nurse while you are there.

After the delivery of the placenta, most hospitals administer a dose of Pitocin, either intravenously or by injection, in order to help the uterus to contract. Inside the uterus, on the site where the placenta was attached, there can be quite a lot of bleeding, and contracting the uterus will aid in controlling this bleeding. After the birth, your uterus will contract to its sixteen- to twenty-week size, and it is extremely important that it remain firm. You can help by massaging your uterus frequently for the first hours after your delivery. Put your hand at the top of the uterus (called the fundus) and make small circles with your hand as you massage, applying pressure. Your fundus is slightly below your navel and will feel like a hard ball beneath your hand.

An important thing to remember is that what may seem to be a huge amount of bleeding to you may not look like heavy bleeding to a nurse or a doctor. There's really no way to prepare you for how much you will, indeed, bleed. In the first one to two days, it is considered normal to change your sanitary napkin every half hour because that napkin is completely soaked.

The flow you experience following childbirth is called *lochia.* It can include clots as well as blood. It's very important that your body pass out these clots, since they can make it difficult for the uterus to contract properly. The flow also has a strange smell (rather like a fishy odor), and over the next few weeks, it goes from a red color to pink and then finally to white before it disappears. You will wear a sanitary belt and napkins, which will be provided by the hospital. When the flow begins to subside, you might want to switch to beltless sanitary pads. You must *not* use tampons. In fact, tampons, tub baths, and sexual intercourse are all prohibited until you see your doctor or midwife for your checkup—usually six weeks after birth. It's also a good idea not to use any deodorant pads, since the perfume in them might be irritating or cause an infection.

To make yourself feel more comfortable, you should change your sanitary pads frequently, especially during the time you are in the hospital. If you find that you have changed a pad and the clean one is soaked within about five minutes or that the blood seems to be creating a puddle in your bed, don't throw the pad away or mop up the flow; call a nurse at once. She'll make sure you aren't hemorrhaging.

When you want to get out of bed for the first time after the baby is born (probably several hours later, or perhaps even one or two hours following delivery), do *not* get up until there is another person present beside you. You probably haven't eaten anything; the blood will have pooled and is going to come out with a rush when you stand; you cannot anticipate how weak you will feel. You can fall and hit your head and really hurt yourself if you try to get up alone. Don't attempt it.

Some people will bleed more than others; there is no set rule. The more children you have, the harder it is for your uterus to contract to normal and the more you will bleed.

One of the biggest problems in the recovery room has to do with urinating. If your bladder is full of urine after the birth, it will take up a lot of space inside you and will push the uterus up and over to the side, where it doesn't have enough room to contract. This can cause problems, because an uncontracted uterus will bleed a great deal. Women can bleed heavily if they have full bladders. Following delivery, many women are scared to go to the bathroom because of their episiotomies and stitches. An added problem is that their bladders have gotten stretched and their sphincter control has been affected; the result is you may not feel the customary urgency you're used to with a full bladder. It is extremely important, though, that you overcome your fears and urinate before leaving the recovery room.

Hospitals will also check your urinary output after the baby's birth; you will be asked to urinate into a bedpan for the first few times. If you can't urinate, you will be catheterized. A catheter will be put in, you will urinate, and it will be removed. Being catheterized can sometimes provide a great deal of relief.

When you leave the recovery room and are admitted to the postpartum floor, in addition to checking your bleeding and your uterus, the nurse will also take your vital signs (blood pressure, temperature, etc.). In the course of future visits, she will examine your stitches and check your breasts.

After delivery, one of the first things some women want is food. You will be permitted to eat within a few hours, unless you've had a Cesarean section, in which case you'll have to wait a day for solid food. You will also be permitted to take a shower. Hospitals will give you soap, soap dishes, towels, and washcloths. You can bring your own soap if you choose, and you must provide your own shampoo and conditioner.

Hospitals will also provide some other necessities that can help you during your stay: sitz baths, hemorrhoid medications, pain medications, nipple cream (if you're nursing), extra pillows to prop you up, ice packs, fruit juice and snacks, and clean nightgowns. Bring your own (preferably old) underwear to put on over your sanitary pad for times when you want to walk around. You'll feel more comfortable wearing panties.

If you do have pain from your stitches, you will want to take some pain medication. Tylenol with Codeine is often given, and it will not be a problem for the baby if you are breast-feeding. It's more important that you be comfortable. If you do not have a bowel movement by the second day, the hospital will also give you some Milk of Magnesia. It's a good idea not to wait too long to see if you go by yourself; constipation can cause problems, especially if you have difficulties with hemorrhoids.

Hemorrhoids can develop during pregnancy, from the weight of the fetus you are carrying, or you may even have had a few problems with them before pregnancy. If this is the case, then delivering the baby will probably have caused them to push out. They can be larger than you've ever had, and consequently more painful. Sitz baths will help to shrink them. (Your sitz bath will also help reduce soreness. Read the instructions for the sitz bath carefully. When used correctly, this portable plastic basin fits over the toilet seat and provides a flow of warm water over your perineal area. A nurse will show you how to use it.) You can also get Anusol suppositories from the nurse to help the hemorrhoids to heal, and small cotton pads soaked in witch hazel (Tucks) are available. Any topical anesthetic that you've been given for your stitches, such as Tronolane cream or Dermoplast spray, will also help with the hemorrhoids.

When lying in bed, prop yourself up on your side if your hemorrhoids make you uncomfortable. But don't avoid walking. Walking will help your stitches and your hemorrhoids. And your Kegel exercises (see Chapter 7) will help as well. If you have a favorite hemorrhoid treatment at home that you've used during your pregnancy, pack it with the things you take to the hospital.

Your episiotomy will also feel sore and painful, depending on how big it is and how many stitches were given. Your perineum will also be sorer if you've had a long second stage of labor or forceps delivery. Don't worry about having the stitches taken out: they won't be. They dissolve and are absorbed into your body. Here too, Kegel exercises will help a great deal, as will walking around. There is also pain medication available, so don't be afraid to ask for some. You will be given a squeeze bottle made of plastic that is commonly called your peri bottle. This is to be filled with warm water and squeezed onto your perineum after you urinate. The flow of warm water feels very good on the sore area. When you shower, don't be afraid to wash the perineal area with a washcloth and soap or your hand, if you prefer. You won't disturb the stitches.

You will experience some contractions in your uterus, called *afterpains*. Frequently, these are felt most sharply during nursing, due to the release of the hormone oxytocin, which is stimulated by the baby's sucking. This is why nursing mothers find that their uteruses contract more rapidly than those of nonnursing mothers. Ask the nurse for some pain medication if the contractions are uncomfortable.

Women who choose to breast-feed will receive some instruction from the nurse on how to begin, but it's a good idea to read up on this subject if it is the method of feeding you have chosen. When you are given the baby for feedings, the most important thing to remember is to relax. Apply some of your prepared-childbirth relaxation techniques. Babies know when you tense up and they tense up. Most women who quit breast-feeding right away do so because they get nervous and very discouraged. There are many books out now that deal with the subject intelligently; it's a worthwhile investment to buy one and bring it to the hospital with you to read between feedings.

Your milk will come in between three and five days following delivery (until then the baby drinks colostrum, the early, premilk substance rich in nutrients), and this is the time when your breasts may feel painful. Make sure you have brought a good brassiere with you—either a real nursing bra or one with strong elastic and firm straps. Many women find it more comfortable to sleep in a bra during the first weeks of nursing, when their breasts are at their heaviest. If you are not nursing, bring a bra that is a bit small and wear it all the time. This will help ease the engorged feeling. You can ask for ice packs or pain medication if binding the breasts doesn't help.

And here, we'd like to say a word to mothers who choose not to breast-feed. Don't feel guilty about your choice. Whatever your reasons, it is up to you to decide. It's more important for you to be relaxed and comfortable with yourself and your new baby than to feel you have to do something you don't want to do simply because you feel the pressure of public disapproval.

Many hospitals now offer mothers the option of

rooming-in with their babies. This means that instead of having your baby cared for in the nursery with the other newborns, the baby lives in your room with you and you care for it. We have a divided reaction to the notion of rooming-in. First of all, rooming-in includes having the baby in the room with you for the entire night. This can be a problem for you, since you've just had a baby and you're going to be exhausted. You'll need your sleep. If your baby is a crier, you probably won't get much rest. Also, the first night following the baby's birth, the baby may still be somewhat mucusy and might need suctioning. Listening to the baby's labored breathing all night could be frightening for you. Rooming-in with the baby also prohibits all visitors except your husband.

The advantages of rooming-in include the fact that since you're the primary care giver (under the nurses' supervision), you will learn very quickly how to take care of your baby. At the same time you'll have the secure feeling that someone is there to correct your mistakes and give you shortcuts and tips on how to do things. It will be easier when the time comes to take the baby home, knowing that you can do everything the hospital does. And you've become familiar with your baby's habits and schedule.

If you would like to try rooming-in, it's a good idea to skip the first night, get your rest, and then proceed with the rooming-in from there. It's also a good idea to find out ahead of time what the hospital's schedule is for allowing the baby in the room with you. You may be surprised to discover that your hospital permits the infant to be in the room with you all day, except for visiting hours, and thus you might not feel that rooming-in is necessary. Check with your doctor or midwife in advance.

If you have had a Cesarean section, your postpartum recovery will be different. You'll experience more discomfort and you will not recover as quickly as a woman who has had a vaginal delivery. There will be pain from the incision, gas, soreness, and fatigue. You'll also have an I.V. for at least a day. General anesthesia will leave you feeling groggy after surgery, and you will feel the pain of the stitches at once. It's advisable to ask for pain medication. You will not be able to breast-feed and bond with the baby right away as you will feel drunk and quite "out of it."

Epidural anesthesia before Cesareans will make it easier for you to bond with the baby and feed the baby, since you'll be numb for up to two hours following surgery. When the numbness starts to wear off, ask for pain medication quickly, since the anesthetic wears away fast. It's important to get up and walk as soon as the doctor and nurses will let you; walking will promote faster healing and recovery. Because you will not be allowed to shower until the stitches are removed, frequent sponge baths will help you feel clean and refreshed. Make an effort to fix your hair and makeup, since you will also be receiving visitors. It's normal to feel sorry for yourself because you've had surgery and other mothers have not. Use this as an excuse to pamper yourself.

When the nurse brings you the baby to hold, let her help you get into a comfortable position. If necessary, take some pain medication before the baby is brought in, so you won't be in pain while holding the baby or feeding it. Don't put the baby down right on top of the area of your incision; put a pillow in your lap first. If you are especially uncomfortable, you may need pain medication often, as much as every three to four hours for the first couple of days. Don't be afraid to ask. We cannot repeat this too often. Your surgery may not make you feel like much of a mother these first few days, but some pain relief might make all the difference.

With Cesareans, the gas pains that follow surgery will abate after a few days, as will the pain of the stitches. By the fifth or sixth day the stitches will come out and you can shower. Some hospitals will send you home; others may keep you for the full seven days. But when you go home, you won't feel like returning to your full schedule and you might need some help for the first week or two. You're entitled to it—after all, you have had major surgery.

But whether you had a vaginal delivery or a Cesarean, look at it this way: you aren't as bad off as the woman who delivered twins, one vaginally and the second by Cesarean section. She had the worst of both worlds!

You should not stock your house with baby supplies before your baby is born. Some women run out during their eighth or ninth month and buy all the baby products on the shelves of the drugstore: cases of newborn disposable diapers, baby lotions, baby creams, ointments, wipes, swabs, and so on. To save yourself a great deal of time and money, it's a good idea to buy as little as possible. First of all, most hospitals give you a going-home kit consisting of samples of many of the products you will use. That way, you can try things out before buying the giant economy size. You may not like all of the products you buy, and it's better to try them than to be stuck with them for months. If your hospital does not hand out freebies, you can always call the drugstore when you arrive home and order a few things right away.

Another reason you may want to wait until after

you've been in the hospital to stock up on supplies is that hospital personnel, the most experienced infant handlers in the world, have many excellent and practical tips about what to use for the baby and definite opinions about what *not* to use. During the bath class at a major New York hospital, the nurse who was demonstrating told the new mothers at each step what she liked to use on the babies. Every time she mentioned a product she thought was unnecessary, or not effective, a collective groan went up from the mothers who had bought a year's supply. You'll find out in the hospital what you really need. And, incidentally, if your baby is a nine- or ten-pound bruiser, which happens more than you think, newborn-size disposable diapers won't be of much use beyond the first few weeks.

This brings us to another important reminder: when you are in the hospital, attend all classes, demonstrations, lectures, and other events arranged for new mothers. Ask questions. The nurses will be your best sources of advice, and with a newborn baby, you'll need (and want) all the advice you can get. Even if you have arranged to have a nurse in your home, it's a good idea to get used to doing things for your baby right away. During a bathing demonstration, you can learn tricks and tips on handling a newborn that you'll use for this and future babies. Don't consider any questions mundane or silly. Ask the nurse how to burp the baby. She'll probably know six different ways your mother never heard of. Learn them all. The nurses can be your best friends during these first anxious days of motherhood.

CHAPTER EIGHTEEN

Welcome to Motherhood: The Postpartum Period

When you leave the hospital, a nurse will carry your baby down to your car and place the baby in your arms for you to take home at last. You will be expected to supply all of the baby's clothes for the going-away outfit, right down to the undershirt. Be sure to pack a receiving blanket and a hat. (Even if it is summer, it's a good idea to cover a newborn's head.) Take your camera along for this precious moment; you'll want to have some pictures. Make sure you yourself have something to wear that *fits.* You won't be your prepregnancy size yet; bring something from your fifth or sixth month.

There are times when you may have to go home without your baby. Premature births, resulting in tiny, underdeveloped babies, or even full-term babies with medical problems, can lead to a mother's being released from the hospital without her baby. This is a very difficult situation and has to be faced with a great deal of strength. You will feel angry because you are different from everyone else, and you may feel guilty, as if the problem was your fault. But there are ways to cope, and one is by knowing that many problems *can* be solved and your baby will be released as soon as it is better.

Premature babies will be put into incubators and cared for until they weigh at least five pounds and are healthy. You are allowed to visit them whenever you like, and you can bond with them even if they are not allowed out of their incubators. Put your fingers into the opening and touch your baby as much as you want. As the baby gets stronger, you may be permitted to hold and feed it. It's important to remember that these tiny babies are often far sturdier than they look, and by the time you do take them home, you will have a lot of experience caring for them and will feel very comfortable.

Neonatal jaundice is a very common condition in newborns, and sometimes, if it is severe enough, the baby will be kept a few extra days until its bilirubin level is normal. Jaundice is caused by an immature liver, which doesn't break down red blood cells properly. This leads to an excess of bilirubin, which the liver cannot cope with, which then circulates throughout the baby's system, causing jaundice. The baby's skin may take on an orange cast as a result. If the bilirubin level is high enough, the doctor may want to keep the baby in the hospital for several more days so as to keep the baby "under the lights." This is a treatment in which phototherapy is used; the baby is kept in an incubator with lights to help break down the excess of bilirubin and help with its reabsorption.

A baby born with other problems, respiratory or digestive or anything that causes the baby to be placed in the intensive-care unit, may be visited twenty-four hours a day. Only parents are allowed this privilege. If this should happen to your baby, it may be extremely difficult for you, but the doctors and nurses caring for your baby will make every effort to explain exactly what is happening. And as difficult as it is to see your baby attached to tubes, it's extremely important for you to treat the baby as *yours.* Talk to the baby, touch it in the incubator, and look forward to the time when the baby will be yours to hold and then to take home. And when the baby is released from the hospital, you should understand that it is no longer considered a "sick" baby. You should not be afraid to take it home and care for it yourself.

You should own one or two basic books on baby care, and you should try to meet and talk to your pediatrician before the birth of your baby. At that time you can discuss his hours and availability, who will cover for him during vacations, what his feelings are about breastfeeding, and whatever else you would like to know about infant and child care. Most doctors are happy to meet prospective parents. And when you bring your baby home from the hospital, feel free to call the doctor if there is any problem. Many pediatricians have established telephone hours, during which you can call them with your questions.

We sometimes call the first six weeks after delivery the fourth stage of labor, because it is a time with its own special demarcations. Your body is still not normal (it takes at least six weeks for your blood volume to return to normal, for your hormones to get back into balance, and for your uterus to return to its normal size), and it is a stage during which physical problems can still arise. It is also a stage of psychological adjustment, when you make the transition to motherhood, when you are getting used to not being pregnant anymore and to having your baby with you. It's important to keep in mind that this emotional transition takes place at a time when you are physically in a state of flux.

No one knows much about the phenomenon known as postpartum blues, but one thing is certain: if you've got them, you think you're the only person in the world going through it. Part of the blue feeling can be attributed to hormone changes, as you come down from the "high" of your pregnant body. But another part stems from cultural guilt. Women think motherhood is instinctive, that it is automatic to feel maternal, to love the baby, to do all the things a "good" mother is supposed to do. But suppose you had a long and difficult labor? You may feel some resentment toward the baby because you feel it's responsible for the pain. What's more, for most of your pregnancy, you've been the one receiving all the attention. All eyes have been focused on you. Now the baby has arrived and is receiving the limelight, and you are the last person who limps down the hall toward the nursery window during visiting hours. Where has all that attention gone? To the baby.

It's common to cry and not know why. In the hospital, many of these feelings are suppressed; you're still "up" from the birth experience. But once you're home, there's a letdown. You look in the mirror and you're appalled by what you see. You feel fat and ugly, your stitches hurt, you can't take a bath in the tub, you're tired, and you're left with a crying baby while your husband goes back to work. You don't feel loved. And your baby doesn't seem to know who you are.

The most important thing to remember about the postpartum blues is, first, that they go away, and second, that you aren't alone. Many women feel this way. We tell people in our childbirth classes to keep in touch with one another after they give birth so they won't feel alone. Here are people in exactly the same situation as you. They'll understand how you feel.

Memo to the Coach

Try to be very understanding. Your wife isn't being a grouch, a bitch, or an unloving mother if she expresses any of these feelings. There are psychological and physiological reasons behind this phenomenon that sometimes occurs. Understand this, be patient, and she will get better. It is not a permanent condition.

However, if you feel so bad that nothing seems to help and this blue feeling continues without a letup, it is a good idea to see someone—your obstetrician or family doctor—to discuss getting professional help.

It will also help if you accept the simple fact that no matter how you feel in the beginning, you are going to grow to love your child. But your feelings may be in turmoil partly from all the work and energy required of you at the start. So get someone to help you: if your husband can't take some time off from work, get your mother or a relative to come by and assist you, or get a nurse for a few days or a week. Then leave the house and do something for yourself. Buy something new to wear, get a manicure, have your hair done.

Most important of all, you and your husband should take some time off from parenthood as a couple. This cannot be stressed enough. Right from the beginning, take at least one night off a week and go out. Before the baby is born, find some baby-sitters, interview them, and be prepared to hire them. It may be very hard to leave your newborn baby with a sitter, but *do it.* If you don't do it right away, the longer you wait, the harder it will be in the future. And even if you can just get away for an hour, even for a walk around the block, get out and be alone with your husband. There's no advice that will help you more during those difficult first months of being parents.

CHAPTER NINETEEN

The Things You Worry About: Questions and Myths

In teaching childbirth classes and in nursing on the labor and delivery floor, we have been asked hundreds of questions by women who have been anxious and fearful about one thing or another. What they ask has been surprising, for it's not the hard questions—"Will my baby be deformed?"—but the seemingly trivial ones—"Can I leave my wedding ring on?"—that we are asked most often.

We have compiled a list of the most frequently asked questions, along with honest answers. You may find some of your worst fears and some of your silliest concerns expressed by other pregnant women in these pages; many of your other questions can be answered by your doctor or midwife or your labor nurse at the hospital. The important thing to remember is what we have stressed throughout this book—*don't be afraid to ask.*

Before we get into the list of questions, we'd like to discuss the biggest fear—usually a secret fear—that every woman has. Most people don't want to think about it, but in some cases, a few cases, the baby does not survive. It is born dead or it has so many problems that it dies soon after birth. This is the hardest thing of all for everyone to face, the parents and the staff alike.

If your baby should die, you will not be placed on the same hospital floor as the other mothers. Many women seem to fear that the most. The mother must have privacy to grieve. She will go through stages, through denial, then guilt over possibly having done something wrong, to anger over why this should be happening to her, to "I don't deserve this," to, finally, acceptance. The doctor will ask for an autopsy unless it is against religious law. An autopsy should indicate if there was a genetic factor involved, and if this is the case, genetic counseling in the future might avoid any further problems with other pregnancies. If a genetic problem is not present, an extremely common cause of full-term stillbirths is a cord accident. The cord may be wrapped around something; it may be occluded or knotted. This causes a great deal of guilt in mothers who think—incorrectly—that frequent exercising or moving around strenuously during their pregnancy may have caused this problem. But one thing to keep in mind about cord accidents is that there is no congenital deformity present that could affect future pregnancies, and the woman can get pregnant again with no worries.

Before another pregnancy is attempted, the woman

should first grieve and come to terms with her loss. Otherwise the pregnancy can lead to other psychological problems.

If this should happen to you, you might feel that the staff is not emotional, that no one really cares. But it is difficult for a staff nurse to deal with death, particularly when death is not expected, and when she works in an environment that is usually so happy. Labor nurses have probably never met the patients who come to their floor, and this can also create some awkwardness. A nurse may feel very bad for a woman who has lost her baby, but she may find it difficult to express her feelings, partly because she is expected to be strong. This often leads to an emotional paradox: "I've cried with a lot of patients I hardly knew," one nurse said. "I couldn't help it. I felt so bad for them. Sometimes crying in front of them was really good. It helped them. There was someone to share their feelings with. But other times crying didn't help them. It made them feel worse, because they wanted me to be strong."

For a nurse, these too are the most trying times, because it can be just as difficult to hold back emotion as it is to show it.

We have divided the most common questions into four subject categories: pregnancy, labor, delivery, and postpartum. And they are followed by a section on myths and misconceptions.

Pregnancy

What if my husband doesn't want to go to childbirth classes?

Try to talk him into going to at least the first class. Make a deal with him: all he has to do is go to one class;

he doesn't have to finish the course. Men are often afraid of "natural" childbirth and of standing by and seeing someone they love in pain while they feel helpless. The first childbirth preparation class may help to dispel these fears, since the teacher is aware that many husbands feel this way.

Your husband may not understand that he can play an enormous part in the birth of his child. Men think having a baby is just the wife's role and there's no place for them, but the teacher will help your husband to understand that he is the person you will need most during childbirth. He'll be with you; you'll have the baby together.

We've changed a lot of people's minds with the first class. We go around the room and ask everyone why they've come, and many men confess that they've been "dragged" to class. Your husband isn't the first to balk, but he won't be the first to change his mind. If the teacher can't talk him into staying for the classes, try to have someone available as a standby coach. Since the first class in the series is usually introductory, your new coach will not miss anything crucial.

What if I have no coach?

You should try to get someone to be your coach—your mother or father, sister or brother, friend, co-worker, anyone you feel you can ask. If you don't have a coach, you can still learn prepared childbirth, although some of it may be more difficult. When you get to the hospital in labor, your nurse will help coach you through your delivery. If you've selected someone to coach you whom you might not want in the delivery room (such as your father), that person can help you through labor and then wait outside, as some prospective fathers choose to do.

When should I call my doctor?

Call immediately if there is something wrong or even if you think there *might* be something wrong. Obstetricians know that pregnant women need attentive care and don't mind those phone calls. Don't hesitate, especially if something out of the ordinary occurs—bleeding, a pain that doesn't go away, breaking your water, or discovering the water is a greenish color.

What if my doctor is in a group practice? How can I make sure I get the doctor I like best for my delivery?

You can't. But you can make it your business to meet *all* the other doctors in the practice sometime during your pregnancy. Then, if one of the doctors you like best or want most is unavailable, at least you'll feel more confident that you know the doctor who's going to deliver your baby.

My doctor practices by himself. How can I be sure I can reach him whenever I need him?

Ask your doctor how his service works (the people who answer his telephone when he is not in the office and who then contact him for you). Find out who covers his practice for him when he is away. Usually it is another doctor on the staff of the same hospital, and your doctor can tell you about him if you are concerned your doctor won't always be available.

My baby is breech, and my doctor says he'll turn my baby around inside me. Will this hurt my baby?

This is called an external version, and it used to be done quite commonly. For the past number of years it has not been used, but it is now coming back again. A doctor will attempt this maneuver toward the end of your pregnancy. You'll sometimes be given Ritodrine, which relaxes your uterus so it won't tense up. They will not give you a relaxant (such as Valium), because they want you to be aware of pain. Pain is an important signal that something is not going right. (If it hurts you, the doctor will stop immediately.) The doctor tries to turn the baby around. Sometimes this works, only to have the baby turn itself back around again to the breech position. Sometimes if it's unsuccessful, the doctor may try it again. It will not hurt the baby if it's done correctly. Your baby's heartbeat will be checked both during the procedure and after.

I'm thirty years old. Should I have amniocentesis? My *doctor says it's not necessary until I'm thirty-five.*

In an amniocentesis, the doctor will use sonography to visualize the fetus. He will then put a needle into your abdomen and through the uterus into the amniotic sac and collect fluid to analyze. By this means, the baby can be checked for genetic abnormalities, most commonly Down's syndrome, which causes mongolism. Neural tube defects can be diagnosed, including spina bifida and genetic diseases such as Tay Sachs. The baby's sex can also be determined.

But having amniocentesis does not guarantee that you

will have a perfectly normal baby. The reason women over thirty-five are told to have the procedure is that the risk of mongolism increases significantly for babies born to women over that age. It isn't necessary before that unless you are a carrier of a specific disease or there is a history of a certain disease in your family. As there is a small risk of aborting following amniocentesis, it's advisable not to have it if there is no real reason.

Will the baby feel what I'm feeling when I'm pregnant?

There is nothing really proven substantially, but it is said that babies in utero hear things and are sensitive to heat, light, and loud noises. It couldn't hurt if you talked to your baby soothingly and experienced it as a person *before* birth.

What if I decide I don't like my doctor in the middle of my pregnancy?

Switch doctors. Your peace of mind is more important than your doctor's feelings. This should not be done lightly, but if your doctor refuses to listen to what you want in a delivery or refuses to consider your options, and you feel pushed into having a natural birth or an epidural or some other procedure, you might want to find someone more responsive to your needs. Judge by your feelings, but give it some time. If you've had one bad visit, remember that the doctor might just be having a bad day.

Is a sonogram dangerous for the baby?

No, as long as it's not done too frequently; it should not be done unless it is indicated. It is a helpful, noninvasive tool used in early pregnancy to date the baby when the dates are not certain, to aid in amniocentesis, to diagnose multiple births, to show the position of the placenta or the position of the baby's head, to discover intrauterine growth retardation (when the baby is not growing well). But it should not be done every week to "see if everything is okay" or simply to find out what sex the baby is. However, if a problem is suspected that calls for sonography, it can be performed as often as once a week, safely.

What if I haven't felt the baby move in a day or so?

From eighteen to twenty weeks on, you should feel your baby move. If it's before that time, don't worry. But after you feel the first movements, you should feel the baby move at least once a day or more. If you don't, tell your doctor immediately.

With all this talk about problems and complications, how do I know if there's a problem going on inside me?

Sometimes you won't know, but in many cases you will feel changes and be aware of differences. You learn to know your pregnant body quite well. You'd be surprised how often women know there is something the matter without any major signs. With some problems, there are signals, such as pain, bleeding, cramping early or mid-pregnancy, swelling of your extremities, a large weight gain in a short period of time, headaches, or dizziness.

Is bleeding during pregnancy always serious?

No, but it is always worth attention. In the first trimester many women experience some bleeding, which may not be significant. More serious bleeding can mean a threatened miscarriage, and when you call your doctor, he'll tell you to get off your feet. There is a fifty-fifty chance that you'll carry the baby to full term. In the third trimester, you may bleed after an examination or after intercourse. Heavy bleeding during this time may mean an abruption or placenta previa. Call your doctor about *any* bleeding.

Why do I always have to give a urine sample when I visit my doctor?

The doctor is checking for sugar, which is an indication of gestational diabetes in the mother. This is common in pregnancy. The level of protein is also checked, an excess of which may indicate toxemia.

What about sex during pregnancy?

If there is any bleeding, the doctor may make you stop for a while. If you're in your third trimester and you bleed from a placenta previa, sex is out. Generally, however, sex doesn't hurt the baby, since the cervix is toward the rear (posterior) and even the deepest penetration does not cause any harm. If it's comfortable for you, sex is usually safe until the end of pregnancy, though some doctors will ask you to stop at thirty-six weeks. Premature labor or other complications may restrict you further. If you have any questions about sex, don't be shy: ask. Your doctor has heard these questions before.

One important thing not often mentioned is to exercise care during oral sex (cunnilingus) throughout pregnancy. In a few cases, air was blown into the woman's vagina and caused an air embolism, which proved extremely dangerous. Do not let any air be blown into the vagina.

I'm prone to urinary tract infections. Is it worse to get one during pregnancy than it is to have one normally?

Yes. Urinary tract infections seem to be associated with premature labor and can be more serious during pregnancy. If you have any signs or symptoms of a UTI during pregnancy such as burning or pain on urination, or back (flank) pain, see your doctor immediately.

If you are prone to these infections, drink lots of fluids, including cranberry juice. Don't take bubble baths. Be sure to urinate before having sex *and* after having sex. The urine taken routinely by your doctor is not checked for infections unless you complain of having symptoms of one.

Everyone's trying to give me advice about my pregnancy, labor, and delivery. What should I do?

Don't listen to anyone. Shut all of it out. How someone else had her baby and experienced her pregnancy and what was right for her isn't necessarily what you will experience and what is right for you.

Labor

What if my water breaks in a public place?

There isn't much you can do if it comes out with a gush. It is a good idea to carry a few sanitary napkins with you during the last two weeks of your pregnancy. If you're going to a theater or a dinner party and you feel concerned about it, bring a small towel. Your water will not necessarily come pouring out; the first signs may be simply a trickle. We jokingly tell our classes to carry a jar of olives or sauerkraut to save embarrassment in a public place. When your water breaks, drop the jar nearby and no one will be any wiser.

A real problem is breaking your water in bed, when you're asleep. This can ruin your mattress. Put a plastic bag under your bottom sheet during your last weeks of pregnancy to prevent this from happening.

What if I freak out in labor and forget what I'm supposed to do?

First of all, this is one of the reasons you have a coach. You can bring the crib notes your childbirth instructor gave you with you to the hospital, or you can make your own notes on your classes or from this book and pack them in your prepared childbirth bag. Second, an observant nurse will help you if you run into difficulty. For example, if you're only dilated one centimeter but you're doing puff-and-blow breathing, she can see the problem and advise you. Listen to her experienced advice and take it.

What if someone brings a bunch of medical students into my room when I'm in labor and I don't want them there?

You have the right to your privacy. You may politely ask them to leave, or simply say (less politely), "Get those medical students out of here."

What if there is no anesthesiologist available and I want an epidural?

If the anesthesiologist is not at the hospital yet or is unavailable, you can be given Demerol by a nurse to help you until one arrives or becomes available.

What if the epidural doesn't work?

They'll try it again. And you can always get Demerol or other pain-relieving drugs if it doesn't work a second time.

Does labor really hurt?

Yes.

What if the nurse insists on giving me an enema and I don't want it?

You can refuse anything; that's part of the patient's bill of rights. But if she persists, don't panic and let it ruin your labor. Having an enema is no big deal.

When should I go to the hospital?

Use your own judgment. Stay at home as long as you can, but you don't want to wait so long that you have to crawl to the hospital on your hands and knees. Some doctors say that if your contractions occur every five minutes for at least one hour, you should go to the hospital. But don't necessarily go by that. If your contractions are five minutes apart but you are still comfortable, stay at home. On the other hand, if the contractions are farther apart than every five minutes but they're very strong, you might want to go to the hospital then. Everyone's labor is different; there are really no hard and fast rules.

However, we can tell you three things that might help: (1) if you can talk during a contraction, it's too early; (2) if you're still smiling, it's too early; and (3) it's not the worst thing in the world to go to the hospital and be sent home.

Are the doctors and nurses really on my side? Will they be nice?

The nurses and doctors are there to help you. And they work very hard to make sure everything goes well.

What should be packed for a snack for my coach?

It's a good idea to take along a thermos of coffee. A sandwich is customary, preferably meat and cheese rather than anything messy or with mayonnaise. Peanut butter and jelly is a good choice. He should also pack a piece of fruit, such as an orange, and something for energy—a brownie or a candy bar.

What is the biggest mistake made by women who come to the hospital in labor?

They pack too much: rolling pins *and* tennis balls in case of back labor, ten extra pillows, eighteen sour lollipops, four negligee sets.

What important item is most commonly left at home when women come to the hospital in labor?

They forget to bring a focal point. Actually, anything can be used as a focal point, but most of them forget to bring something along. They don't remember that on the labor floor, the only magazines we have are medical journals, so unless they want to focus on a picture of a uterus or a closeup of a trichomonas infection under a microscope, they're out of luck. B.Y.O. is the best policy.

Delivery

Is the Leboyer method better?

The Leboyer method refers to what is known as gentle birth, or birth without violence. The room is darkened, the noise level is reduced, the baby is placed right on the mother's chest, the clamping of the cord is delayed, and the baby is placed into a warm bath.

Since the baby needs stimulation to breathe, and the entry into the world often helps with respiration, the Leboyer method isn't necessarily the best way to deliver a baby. A warm bath as well may not be the best thing for a newborn infant whose temperature regulation doesn't work too well. This can lead to unpleasant side effects in some babies.

Leboyer births are not necessarily best for the health and well-being of the baby, but if you are interested in the procedure, read up on it. Then talk to your doctor and see if your hospital provides the facilities for it. If you can't do it, your baby is not going to suffer. Babies born in any delivery room are treated gently and are given to the mothers very quickly.

Remember that if there is anything at all wrong with

the baby or if the baby's Apgar scores are not high, the Leboyer method may not be used.

What if I scream?

You won't be the first—or the last. No one will be shocked by it. If you get out of control, you'll probably be offered some pain relief. No one is going to leave you all alone in a room, screaming.

What if my doctor can't get there on time?

If you are having such a rapid delivery that your doctor cannot arrive on time, chances are everything is going very well. But in case of a blizzard or traffic jam or toll collector's strike, in a teaching hospital, residents will always be there. In any hospital, there will be another attending physican available. Also, remember that nurses are qualified to deliver babies. We have, many times, and everything has been fine.

What if I can't get there on time?

It's very unusual with a first baby not to get to the hospital on time, since first labors usually take quite a while. But if you are in a car and you know you can't make it, tell the person driving to pull over. Do not keep driving if the baby is coming. You'll need someone's help with the delivery, and, most important of all, you need to calm down.

The person with you should follow these simple instructions: he or she should place one hand on the perineum to avoid any tearing. Then tell the woman to push gently and help guide the baby out as she pushes. The baby will turn its head to the side naturally, and the shoulders can then be delivered. The rest of the baby will simply slide out. The cord does not have to be cut and tied. Leave the baby attached to the mother and wrap it in a blanket or, if there is none, some newspaper. If the afterbirth should come out, the biggest concern is bleeding. The mother should rigorously massage her belly after the placenta delivers.

When you feel delivery is near and you're not close to the hospital, blowing out as you breathe—puffing—can help control the urge to push and may enable you to get there on time.

What if something is wrong with my baby? Will they show it to me?

It is rare that birth defects occur without advance knowledge. If problems arise during delivery, you may be put to sleep for the baby's birth. If it should happen that you are awake, and that the problem is a surprise, the doctor will hand the baby to a nurse, and will deliver the afterbirth and make sure you are not bleeding. Then we'll come and talk to you. No one will hand you a baby with a problem without discussing it with you first.

However, some major problems, such as Down's syndrome or severe cardiac defects, are not always noticeable immediately at birth. Some heart problems are not manifested for a few hours after birth. And many Down's syndrome babies look quite normal at birth.

If my baby isn't alive, will I have to be awake for the birth?

In the case of a stillbirth that is known ahead of time, you'll be heavily sedated.

If my baby dies at birth or is born dead, can I still hold it and see it?

Yes.

If I'm in labor a long time and don't deliver, will my doctor want to give me a Cesarean section?

Yes. An extremely long labor that doesn't progress can be very dangerous for both the mother and the baby. If you've trusted your doctor throughout your pregnancy, you have to be prepared to accept the decisions he or she may have to make at the end of your pregnancy. You will not, however, be wheeled into the operating room without being asked. Your doctor will explain everything to you ahead of time, including the reasons for the surgery.

I've been seeing a midwife throughout my pregnancy, but because of the baby's position, I'll probably need a Cesarean section. Who will deliver my baby?

Sometime during your pregnancy, you've met with a doctor who will most likely be the one to perform the surgery. In birthing centers in hospitals, midwives usually introduce you to the doctor on call. In maternity centers associated with hospitals, you have to go to the hospital to meet the doctor who will be treating you.

In an emergency, however, you might not know the doctor. But midwives do prepare you for the possibility that you may need a doctor.

What if I don't want an episiotomy?

Discuss this with your doctor. Sometimes an episiotomy is not a matter of choice. The size of your baby and the size of your perineum will determine whether you have one or not.

How will I feel after my baby is delivered?

Exhausted—but terrific. There's a natural "high" after delivery that makes you forget your fatigue and your aches and pains.

Do you get attached to your patients and care about what happens to them and to their babies?

Yes!

Postpartum

Will my stitches bother me a lot?

Yes, but the amount of trouble they'll give you will vary. Most women who have episiotomies do feel some discomfort afterwards, depending on the size and location of their stitches. Those women troubled by hemorrhoids will find that their condition adds to the pain in that area. Your hemorrhoids are always far worse after delivery. There are things you can do following childbirth to relieve some of this discomfort: you can put ice on the area right away, which will be soothing and will help reduce the swelling; you can take frequent sitz baths; a local anesthetic spray such as Dermoplast works adequately; and there are cushions shaped like doughnuts to sit on. Within a day of delivery you should be doing your Kegel exercises and walking, both of which promote blood flow to the perineum, helping it to heal faster. The nurses will check you frequently to see if your stitches are inflamed, but if you experience a good deal of discomfort, tell the nurse or doctor at once.

A friend of mine said she felt she couldn't stop shaking after the baby was born. Does this happen often?

Yes, it can. Shaking after the baby is born can result from the sudden blood loss following delivery as the body attempts to redistribute the remaining blood. It can also come from a sympathetic nervous system response, that is, an involuntary reaction to the shock of delivery. It does not last long, perhaps up to an hour, and is more common for women who have had epidurals.

Will I have trouble urinating after the baby's birth?

Some women do. This is associated more closely with an epidural, as the nerves supplying the bladder and sphincter muscles are not entirely under control following anesthesia. It can also be normal in a vaginal delivery. Many women do find it difficult to void because they're afraid to urinate; they're afraid it will burn. But it doesn't. It's important to pass urine following delivery because otherwise you'll be catheterized, which is not a pleasant alternative.

Will they feed me after I have the baby?

In some hospitals, you will have to wait an hour after delivery in case of excessive bleeding, because then you might need surgical care and it would not be a good idea to have eaten. Most women, however, do not bleed profusely, and in other hospitals, such as ours, you will be fed sooner. There is no reason why you cannot eat within a couple of hours, unless you've had a Cesarean section.

Does the hospital give you anything for the baby when you go home?

In many hospitals, you will receive a box of sample-size baby-care products. This might include disposable diapers, formula, cotton swabs, baby ointment, baby powder, and baby oil. Please remember that you are not given any clothing for the baby and must bring a going-home outfit to the hospital.

Am I going to feel gross for the first few days after the baby comes?

Right after delivery you will. But you really won't or shouldn't by the time you go home. You'll be allowed to shower fairly soon after delivery, which will help. The sanitary napkin, which is bulkier than the pads you may normally use, may make you feel gross because you're unaccustomed to it. Also, you won't be back to your normal weight right away and your body will be undergoing a number of rather severe hormonal changes, so you won't be as glowy as you were when you were pregnant. But the feeling of being out of shape and sore is only temporary.

What can I do to help myself feel more attractive?

Take frequent showers and keep yourself squeaky clean during the first weeks after the baby's birth. Have your hair done: cut, change, perm, or color your customary style. Put on makeup no matter how hurried and tired you feel each day. Get to an exercise class as soon as your doctor allows you, but don't diet if you're breast-feeding. And although you can't have sex with your husband for the first weeks, you can still be sexual toward each other. That will make you feel closer to your old self.

Myths and Misconceptions

We've decided to include some of the most commonly believed myths so you won't feel you have to waste any of your precious time during your pregnancy worrying about things your grandmother or your mother or your sister-in-law told you to worry about. These include the following:

If I have a lot of heartburn, the baby is going to be very hairy.

If I carry very low and mainly in the front, I'll have a boy. If I carry high and more toward the back, I'll have a girl.

If I add some of my morning urine to a few spoons of Drano, I can tell what the baby's sex will be by the color it turns.

If the heart rate of the fetus is fast, it's a girl. If the heart rate is slow, it's a boy.

If I reach up to a high shelf or stretch to the top of a closet, my baby will be born with the cord around its neck.

As long as I'm nursing, I won't get pregnant again.

I'm only allowed a maximum of two Cesarean sections.

If I've had one C section, I have to have another.

It's better to have a premature baby born in the seventh month than in the eighth month.

If I see ugly things during my pregnancy, my baby will turn out ugly.

Eating fresh strawberries during pregnancy causes red, blotchy birthmarks on the baby.

None of these statements is true. Heartburn has nothing to do with hair, and the shape of abdomens, heart rates, and the color of Drano and urine do not predict the sex of the child you're carrying. Reaching up for things on shelves doesn't cause the cord to wrap around the baby; this can occur in any pregnancy, but no one knows why. By reading this book you know that having a Cesarean does *not* dictate future Cesarean births, and there's no limit to the number of Cesareans you can have; we had one case in which a woman had eleven! Premature babies are better off the longer they are in the uterus. And what you see, eat, and do during pregnancy will in no way affect the way your baby looks.

But as far as your fears, misconceptions, and worries are concerned, you don't have to feel foolish if these things (and others like them) trouble you. You're not alone. We've never known a pregnant woman who didn't worry about something. There's a real sense of the unknown about pregnancy. You're carrying a baby you know nothing about, a person whose identity is a mystery to you.

The best antidote to all that worry is your own common sense. We cannot emphasize enough the importance of trusting your own emotions and feelings. If you feel something isn't right, call your doctor. If it seems to you that something you might like to do won't be good for the baby, don't do it. You know about as much as anyone about your own pregnancy.

Nursing on the labor and delivery floor has given us, above all else, a sense of how different each woman's pregnancy is from every other woman's. And because every woman's is different, there's no way to say one thing that will encompass all of them. We have to counsel women to trust their judgment and to listen to what their bodies and their heads tell them.

And above all, remember what you're here for; remember your ultimate goal. When you see that baby, everything will seem worth it—the varicose veins, stretch marks, nausea, heartburn, water retention. Most will be gone, or forgotten, by the time you take the baby home.

But people lose perspective when they're pregnant. They feel sorry for themselves: they're big; they're uncomfortable; they can't find a place to put themselves. We hear all of this in our classes. It's as if women forget that pregnancy is temporary.

The other important thing we want you to remember is this: labor is a great equalizer. On the labor and delivery floor, celebrities and movie stars, society queens and models, go through labor just like you and me. They scream. They yell. They curse. They sweat. They lose control. They get it back. Just like you and me.

So there it all is, the sum total of our experience. We've told you everything we know. *Now* go out there and have your baby. You're on your own, but you won't be alone. You'll have lots of support, and you'll get through it just fine.

And the best thing of all is that your baby doesn't care how you do in labor. He or she is not coming out into the world to give you a report card on how you did. Whatever happens, the baby will love you. And isn't that what this is all about?

We wish you all the very best of luck.

BIRTHING GLOSSARY

ABRUPTION The peeling off or premature separation of either part of the placenta or the whole placenta from the uterine lining.

ACTIVE LABOR The second phase of the first stage of labor, in which the cervix dilates up to four centimeters.

AFTERBIRTH The placenta, umbilical cord, and membranes that are delivered approximately five minutes after the baby is born. (This is considered the third stage of labor.)

AFTERPAINS Contractions of the uterus following delivery that help prevent bleeding and restore the uterus to its normal size.

AMNIOCENTESIS The procedure in which a small amount of amniotic fluid is removed with a needle from the uterine cavity for the purpose of diagnostic tests.

AMNIOTOMY The artificial rupture of the membranes.

AMNIOTIC FLUID The waterlike liquid that surrounds the baby contained within the amniotic sac; its function is to regulate temperature, protect the baby from trauma, and provide for symmetrical growth.

ANALGESIC A central nervous system depressant that lowers the threshold of pain.

ANAL SPHINCTER MUSCLE A circular muscle that controls the opening to the anus.

ANESTHETIC A local anesthetic induces a loss of feeling in the area in which it is injected. A regional anesthetic induces a loss of feeling in the entire area below the level at which it is injected. A general anesthetic induces a loss of consciousness.

ANTEPARTUM The period from conception to delivery.

APGAR SCORE A determination of fetal well-being based on five criteria: heart rate, respiration, tone, reflex, and color. The Apgar score is given at one and five minutes after birth.

BACK LABOR A type of labor characterized by the woman's feeling contractions in her lower back rather than in her abdomen due to the position of the baby's head pressing against her spine.

BILIRUBIN A pigment produced during the breakdown of red blood cells. It can color the skin yellow when the liver is immature; elevated levels are present in neonatal jaundice.

BIRTH CANAL Another term for the vagina.

BLOODY SHOW A vaginal discharge, consisting of a combination of mucus and blood, that is dislodged from the cervix and passed by the pregnant woman around the time of labor or shortly before labor begins.

BRADYCARDIA A slow heart rate. In a fetus and newborn this is less than 120 beats a minute.

BRAXTON HICKS CONTRACTIONS Irregular, erratic contractions of the uterus that can occur throughout the pregnancy. Later in the pregnancy they can increase in frequency and intensity and can sometimes begin the effacement of the cervix. "False labor" is often the result of Braxton Hicks contractions. They are named after an English gynecologist.

BREECH A position of the baby in which the buttocks or feet emerge first.

CATHETERIZATION Insertion of a tube into the bladder to empty it.

CENTIMETERS The measurement used to describe the dilatation of the cervix. One "finger" is two centimeters. Two and a half centimeters is an inch. When you are ready to deliver, you are dilated ten centimeters.

CEPHALOPELVIC DISPROPORTION A condition in which the pelvis is too small to allow the baby's head to mold into it. When this occurs, a Cesarean section is usually required for delivery.

CERVIX The necklike lower part of the uterus that opens during labor to allow the baby's head to pass.

CESAREAN SECTION The delivery of a baby surgically through an incision in the abdominal and uterine walls.

COLOSTRUM The yellowish, rich-in-protein liquid produced by the breasts before the milk comes in.

CONTRACTION The regular tightening and shortening of uterine muscles; in labor they occur rhythmically and cause effacement and dilatation.

CROWNING When the largest part of the baby's head appears in the perineum.

DILATATION The gradual opening of the cervix to allow the baby to pass; it is caused by uterine contractions in labor and is measured in centimeters.

DOWN'S SYNDROME A genetic defect causing mental retardation in an infant; sometimes called mongolism.

EDEMA A fluid accumulation in tissue causing swelling. This is most common in the legs and feet during pregnancy.

EFFACEMENT The thinning and shortening of the cervix.

EFFLEURAGE A light, circular massaging of the abdomen sometimes used during labor by the mother.

ENEMA A procedure in which fluids are introduced into the rectum to cause the bowels to empty.

ENGAGEMENT When the presenting part of the baby enters into the pelvis; also called lightening or dropping.

EPIDURAL A regional anesthesia that is administered by injection through a small catheter into the space in front of the lower spine. This produces pain relief throughout the body from that level down.

EPISIOTOMY A small incision made in the perineum to enable the baby to pass more freely. This is done when the baby is crowning.

EXTERNAL VERSION An attempt late in pregnancy by the doctor to turn a breech position baby around by external manipulation with his hands.

FALSE LABOR Regular or irregular contractions of the uterus that do not dilate the cervix, sometimes mistaken for the first stage of labor.

FETAL ANOMALIES Another term for birth defects.

FETAL DISTRESS A condition in which the baby's flow of oxygen is threatened.

FETAL HEART The baby's heartbeat, usually heard through an ultrasonic device on the abdomen or by stethoscope. The normal range is 120 to 160 beats per minute.

FETAL MONITORING Keeping track of the baby's heartbeat by using an electronic device either internally or externally.

FETUS The developing baby in the uterus from the twelfth week of pregnancy to delivery.

FIRST STAGE OF LABOR The stage that begins at the onset of regular uterine contractions and ends at full dilatation (ten centimeters).

FOLEY CATHETER A rubber tube inserted into the bladder to drain urine from the body.

FORCEPS DELIVERY Delivery of a baby with the assistance of an instrument that is placed on either side of the baby's head. The forceps are used during the second stage of labor when a woman is having difficulty pushing out the baby on her own.

FULLY DILATED The complete dilatation of the cervix to ten centimeters.

FUNDUS The thickest, most muscular portion of the uterus; the top of the uterus, where the contractions originate.

HEMORRHAGE Excessive bleeding.

HEMORRHOIDS Swollen blood vessels around the rectum.

HYDROCEPHALY A congenital abnormality in which excess cerebrospinal fluid accumulates in the baby's brain, causing an enlargement of the head.

HYPERTENSION High blood pressure.

HYPOTENSION Low blood pressure.

INDUCTION Starting labor through the use of Pitocin, a man-made version of the hormone oxytocin, which stimulates uterine contractions.

INTRAMUSCULAR INJECTION The injection of a medication into the muscle.

INVOLUTION The process in which the uterus returns to a prepregnant state after childbirth; this usually takes six weeks.

ISOLETTE A small baby bed enclosed by glass or plastic in which a baby's temperature can be regulated carefully by using a built-in warming device set by a thermostat and through whose sides the baby can be watched closely.

I.V. The intravenous infusion of sterile fluid for the purpose of nutrition, hydration, or medication.

JAUNDICE A common condition in newborn babies in which the skin is a yellowish color due to the buildup of bilirubin caused by an immature liver.

KEGEL EXERCISES Exercises in which the vaginal muscles are tightened and relaxed.

LANUGO The downy hair that covers the fetus and that can sometimes be present, in small amounts, at birth.

LATENT PHASE The first phase of the first stage of labor, in which the cervix dilates up to four centimeters.

LEBOYER METHOD Another theory of delivery in which the lights in the room are dimmed, the noise level is reduced, the baby is placed on the mother's chest immediately, the clamping of the cord is delayed, and the baby is placed in a warm bath. The method is named after Frederick Leboyer, the doctor who invented it.

LIGHTENING Another term for engagement.

LOCHIA The discharge of blood, mucus, and tissue from the uterus that follows birth; it can last for several weeks.

MECONIUM The baby's first bowel movement, which is thick, tarry, and dark green or black; it can be passed in utero before birth.

MINI PREP A partial shaving of the perineum.

MOLDING The shaping and overlapping of the bones in the baby's skull that allows for passage through the birth canal.

MUCUS PLUG A clot of mucus and blood that blocks the cervical canal and can be discharged during labor; also referred to as bloody show.

NONSTRESS TEST A test that monitors the baby's heartbeat and correlates it with the baby's movements.

OXYTOCIN A hormone produced by the pituitary gland that stimulates uterine contractions.

PELVIS The bones that form a girdle around the hips.

PERI BOTTLE A plastic squeeze bottle you receive in the hospital after delivery; squeezing warm water on your perineum after urinating helps the healing of the episiotomy.

PERINEUM The area of tissue between the vagina and the rectum.

PITOCIN Synthetic oxytocin.

PLACENTA The organ that grows on the wall of the

uterus during pregnancy. It provides for the baby's nutrition, oxygenation, and excretion. Also called afterbirth.

PLACENTA PREVIA A condition in which the placenta implants low inside the uterus and partially or completely covers the cervical opening.

POSTMATURE A baby in an overdue pregnancy at forty-two weeks or more.

POSTPARTUM A period of approximately six weeks after the birth of the baby.

PREECLAMPSIA An illness that can occur during pregnancy in which the woman develops high blood pressure, edema, and protein in the urine. Also known as toxemia.

PREMATURE A baby born before the thirty-seventh week of pregnancy or one that weighs less than five pounds at birth.

PRENATAL Before the birth of the baby.

PRESENTING PART The part of the baby that comes out first during delivery.

PRODROMAL LABOR Contractions at the beginning of labor that efface the cervix. This does not occur in some labors.

PUDENDAL BLOCK A form of anesthesia given by

injection into the pudendal nerve which numbs the entire bottom; used for low forceps deliveries.

ROOMING-IN When the baby stays in the mother's hospital room after birth instead of in the nursery and she, rather than the nurses, takes care of the baby.

SECOND STAGE OF LABOR The time from complete dilatation until birth.

SITZ BATH A small plastic bowl with a seat that is filled with continuously running warm water and is used to help heal episiotomy stitches and hemorrhoids.

SONOGRAPHY The use of ultrasonic waves to get a picture of the fetus during pregnancy; this is used for a variety of diagnostic reasons, including locating the fetus during amniocentesis.

SPINA BIFIDA A congenital defect in the walls of the spinal canal.

STILLBIRTH The delivery of a baby that has died in utero.

TACHYCARDIA A fast heart rate; in the fetus and the newborn, this is over 160 beats per minute.

TAY SACHS DISEASE An inherited genetic disease mainly occurring in Eastern European Jews and their descendants.

TERM The complete cycle of the pregnancy, usually considered to be thirty-seven weeks.

THIRD STAGE OF LABOR The time from the birth of the baby until the placenta is expelled.

TOXEMIA Another term for preeclampsia.

TRANSITION The last part of the first stage of labor, when the cervix dilates from seven to ten centimeters.

VERNIX The cheesy substance that covers the skin of the fetus in utero to protect it from the effects of the amniotic fluid on its skin.

APPENDIX:

FOUR IMPORTANT CHECKLISTS

The Fundamentals of Technique

1. Choose a comfortable position.
2. Find a focal point.
3. Take deep cleansing breaths.
4. Practice verbal and nonverbal cues.

What to Pack for the Labor Room

1. Sour lollipops
2. Tennis balls
3. Talcum powder

4. Lip balm
5. Mouth spray
6. Sweat socks
7. Pillow
8. Picture or object for focal point
9. Washcloth
10. Bands, barettes for hair
11. Snack for the coach
12. Crib notes
13. Telephone numbers and dimes
14. Camera
15. Champagne
16. Hot water bottle or dry ice pack

What to Pack for Your Hospital Stay

1. Robe
2. Slippers
3. Socks
4. Nightgowns
5. Underpants
6. Going-home outfit
7. Bras
8. Cosmetics
9. Makeup
10. Outfit for the baby to wear on the trip home
11. Books
12. Pad and pen
13. Radio, bedside clock, tape cassettes and recorder
14. Polaroid camera

The Ten Commandments for Coaches

1. *Be encouraging:* Speak in a calm, reasonable, and gently encouraging voice even though the person you're addressing may be screaming and flailing around.
2. *Be brief:* During active labor and transition, keep conversation to a minimum. At times, a word or two is best. However, during early labor, chatting is okay.
3. *Be gentle:* Your touch should be both light and gentle. Your goal is to soothe, not to distract. Don't break her concentration.
4. *Be responsible:* Learn all the techniques along with her; it's part of your job. You must make sure she is doing things correctly.
5. *Be conscientious:* Take all of this seriously; it's not a joke. When labor starts, you'll be glad you did.
6. *Be supportive:* Stand behind her, no matter what she decides. Don't make her feel guilty or discouraged. If she needs help or pain relief, see that she gets it. Remember, you're not going through labor; she is.
7. *Be calm:* No matter what happens, don't panic. If people are moving fast, if events seem unfamiliar, stay cool. The staff knows what to do; she'll need you to be steady and in control.

8. *Be there:* Try not to leave her side, especially from transition through delivery. Change into a scrub suit ahead of time; go to the bathroom and have your cigarette break earlier. Your presence and encouragement are needed most here.

9. *Be open:* Childbirth isn't just "yucky"; share this experience together. The birth of a baby is really quite wonderful.

10. *Be proud:* Coaches are essential in prepared childbirth; your job is extremely important and quite tough. She couldn't do it (as well) without you!

INDEX